# Bodylife

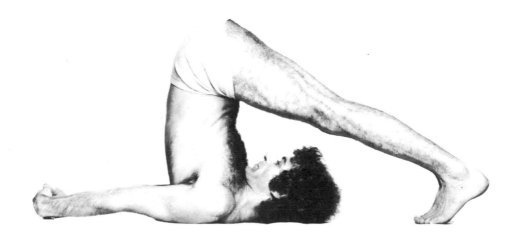

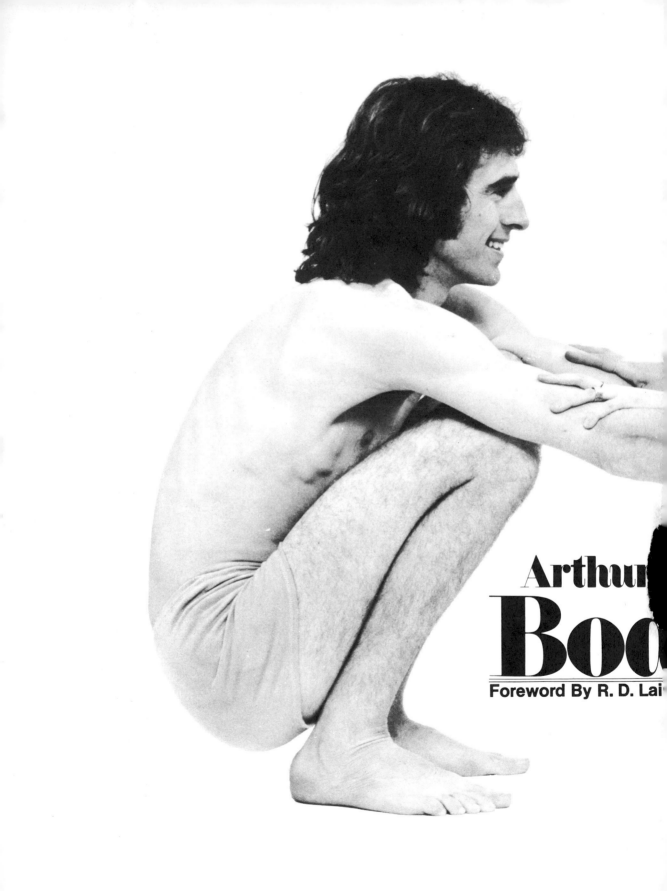

# Arthu~
# Boo

**Foreword By R. D. Lai~**

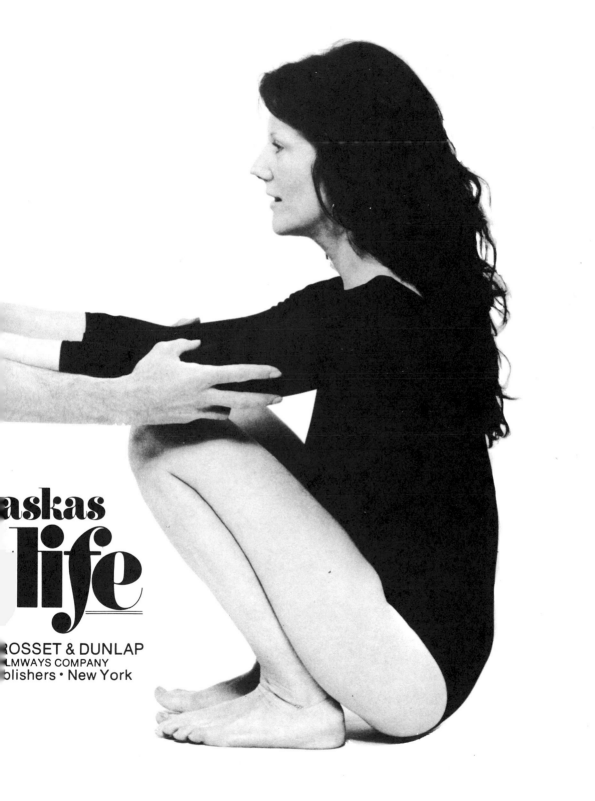

askas
life

GROSSET & DUNLAP
FILMWAYS COMPANY
Publishers • New York

*To Ronnie Laing, who gave me*
*the fortune of a challenge*

Photographs by
  Rosemary Adams
  Heini Schneebeli
  Dorothee v. Greiff
  Drawings by Janet Balaskas

First published in 1977 in Great Britain by Sidgwick & Jackson Limited
Copyright © 1977 by Arthur Balaskas
Library of Congress catalog card number: 77-79106
ISBN 0-448-14500-6

First American edition 1977
Printed in the United States of America

# Contents

Foreword by R. D. Laing/7

Introduction/8

**Part 1**

1 Your body is your friend and home/11
2 Possessing your body and proprioception/12
3 Making friends with your pain/17
4 Knowing your body through touch/20
5 Bones/30
6 Joints/34
7 Muscles/42
8 Blood/47
9 Breathing/50
10 Direct relaxation/53

**Part 2**

11 The ground rules: questions and answers/59
12 Flexibility/62

Neck and shoulder movements
Hip joint, knee and ankle movements
Rotating of trunk
Bending back or extending trunk
Hands, wrists and feet

13 Balance/125

Neck–shoulder balance
Head balance
Elbow balance
Hand balance

14 Resting/139
15 Your movement programme/140
16 Practising with two or more/144
17 Fun for children/150
18 Movements for pregnant women/159
19 Backache/166
20 Exercises in the office/178
21 How people benefit/184
22 A look at yoga and meditation/188

Index/192

# FOREWORD BY Dr R.D.LAING

This book is about joints and muscles: about stiff joints, tense muscles, constricted and jerky movements. And it is about how we may go about loosening our joints, relaxing our muscles, and moving freely. Wouldn't it be nice to be lithe and supple again. Remember?

It is clearly written and the method is simple. But oh, that it were as easy as it is simple! This book makes it as easy for *you* as it can, but only you can stop *dis*easing yourself.

We see stiff, jerky people everywhere. It may come as a shock to realise that we are them. It is all too easy to become a functional cripple without noticing. Can I shake my head? Can I flutter my fingers and wiggle my toes? Do my joints creak if they move at all?

This book sounds the alarm. It emphasizes that we may become oblivious of our body feelings. When I look at my body from the outside, it is still there, but it may have disappeared years ago as a real alive experience from within.

As we become numb, we are numbed to our own numbness. The less we care, the less we care about caring less. We stiffen, harden, shrivel, become bent, but can't bend, twist, run, hop, dance and sing, walk, sleep, even. We lapse painlessly into the complacent ease of bodily vacuity. We may have to think about it before we realise how unfamiliar this most intimate of all our feelings may be. We cannot 'tune' our bodies without being able to 'hear' them. This book is full of tips, hints, and clues on how to tune into, and attend to, our body feelings, and on how to respond appropriately to them.

It can be recommended both to the venturesome and the cautious. To the venturesome, it is the direct approach. Stick to the straight and narrow and you will have many thrills and make many discoveries on the way. But keep at it, and the *real* rewards will come, step by step, reliably, plainly, definitely, actually. *Then* you can relax.

If you feel you would like to get into your body, but feel too proud to admit it, or too ashamed to confess it, or that it's a waste of time, or self-indulgent, or too difficult, or that it's too late, you're past it, then this book comes as a breath of fresh air, blowing these cobwebs away.

And if you have got the message, and want to get on with it, here is an invitation to the adventure of bodylife.

Arthur Balaskas has written this book out of his own successful struggles with these difficulties. It should hearten the disheartened. The path is strewn with thorns, but they turn to roses as one treads upon them.

**R. D. Laing** 9 November 1976

# Introduction

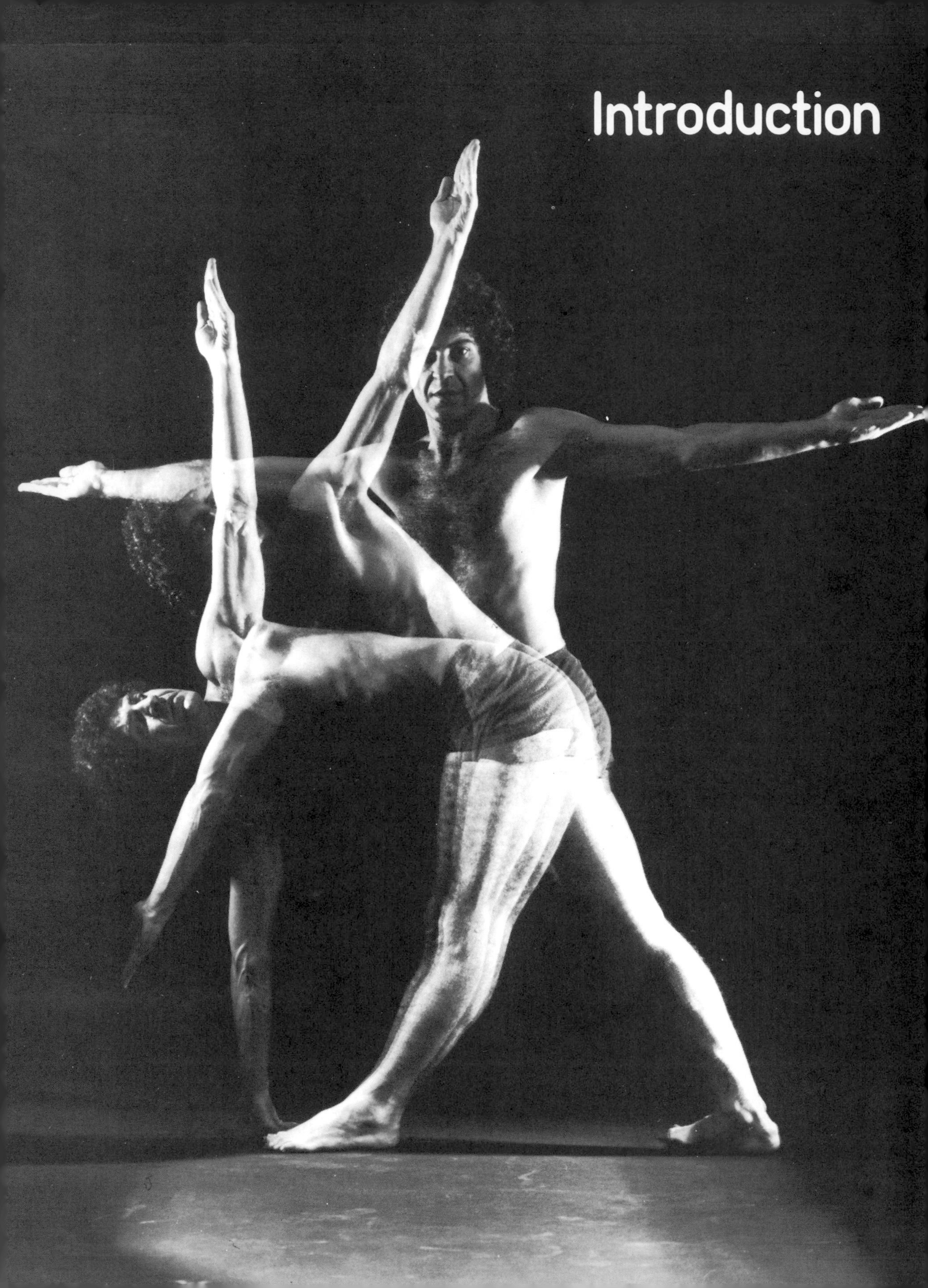

At the age of thirty I made the painful discovery that I suffered from the following difficulties – an exaggerated lower back curve, bent upper back, sunken chest, rounded shoulders and a poorly balanced head. In addition, I experienced what are called migraine headaches, sinusitis, abdominal pains, nausea and tension pains in my back, neck and shoulders.

Through the observation of a friend, R. D. Laing, I became aware of myself as a person with an unnatural posture and restricted movements at most joints. Although I had been active in sports most of my life I realized that my body movements were extremely limited. I was a prisoner of my own muscles and could not touch my toes with my knees straight, nor could I raise my arms to the vertical without difficulty and without arching my back. The movements of my head were very strained and I could not turn to the left or right more than about sixty degrees. I assumed that my skill and activity in sports would have given me bodily well-being. They had, in so far as they had taught me to utilize my body as a co-ordinated unit. But sports could not give me general suppleness at the joints. And this, I have learned, is crucial to a healthy, alive body. Creating suppleness at my joints became my challenge.

My growing awareness of this took me on a journey of self-discovery, an exploration of the bone, joint and muscle operations of my body. I found no single text that gave me insight into these matters and that covered the ground of what seemed to me to be important. I searched for what I needed in the disciplines of yoga, meditation, tantra, psychology, anatomy, physiology and other fields. This book is the result of that search.

Theory must stand the test of practice. In this book what I have written is what I, and later my students, have experienced. I have assembled here, I believe, the fundamentals of a method of recovering body-sense and creating movement at the joints. This knowledge and these techniques should be ours naturally, but, perhaps because of their simplicity, they are generally overlooked or not considered important. The title 'bodylife' condenses the self-evident facts that life is movement, life is sensation. To increase sensation and movement is to increase life. Of all the sensations and movements of our bodies those of our joints are most susceptible to change through personal effort.

Stiffness at the joints relates to restricted actions of the body as a whole and consequently poor body balance or posture. Among the other effects of restricted movement at the joints is loss of energy. This loss is progressive, arising from the conflict between the way your body is built to operate and the way in which it actually operates. The body is constructed in a certain way, mediated by the most efficient use of joints and muscles. Restriction in any part affects the entire system.

I learned to view our physical actions in terms of their common basis: their orientation of our bodies in space. From this viewpoint our smallest movements are part of the dance we perform throughout our lives. It could be called the dance of our changing equilibrium. Our movements are part of the vast continuum of motion in which we live spaced by the resting states that are postures.

We need an awareness of how our own bodies work and do not work. It became clear to me that a lack of consideration and attention to one's body results in impaired functioning, frequently of a minor yet chronic nature. All these impairments are not going to yield to any treatment until the body situation which has caused them is cleared up. Taking drugs for neck and back pain, for instance, may sometimes be necessary, but only after the preconditions of restricted movement at joints and excessive muscle tension have been examined and cleared will there be any lasting improvement. Drugs can only temporarily help a condition that you are perpetuating posturally by limited movement. I have found that creating movement at joints does away with a host of seemingly unrelated conditions.

This book and its techniques are for those who wish to improve their range of movements at body joints, to increase balanced uprightness, to change the shape of their physique and to better the general muscle tone of their bodies. Just as our potential in this machine age has been multiplied many times by the very machines we have created, so we can multiply our personal potential by applying equal intelligence and effort to our own mechanism.

In my own case, simply creating movement and thus sensation at body joints has resulted in many benefits. I now have far more energy, better concentration and attention and feel better equipped to deal with sickness. The shape and posture of my body have changed and my body has become a source of pleasure to me. Increased body-sense has brought me a feeling of rootedness or centring with a noticeable loss of self-consciousness. I have made friends with pain and through this process dissolved or let go much hidden pain. My breathing has deepened. I have a better skin colour and generally feel fitter. I have learned to know my body better and to possess it in a way I never thought possible. The more efficient my body becomes the more it generates confidence, and for the first time health or bodily well-being has become a personal responsibility. But the experience of awakening from a lifelong nightmare of physical discomfort is impossible to describe. Remaining constantly stiff seems to me far more unpleasant than particular instances of stiffening up.

# PART 1    1 Your body is your friend and home

Your body is like a friend with whom you spend your life. You live with it, eat with it, relax with it, move with it, sense with it, sleep with it, all your life. This being so, you may as well learn its strengths and weaknesses and learn to co-operate and work with it. If you give it the time and attention it deserves you will be surprised what a good friend and home your body can be.

Some bodies are better friends than others, and that is because they are more alive. How can you tell? Here are some of the signs.

Breathing is deep.
Eyes sparkle.
Muscle tone is good.
Skin colour is bright.
The body is warm.
The voice seems to come from low down.
The set of the jaw is straight.
The shoulders are hanging, broad and light.
The alignment of the backbone produces shallow curves.
Body movements are easy and wide in range.

A person with such a rhythmic and relaxed body is energetic, awake, uninhibited in self-expression and able to respond freely and spontaneously.

Most people, however, are not fluid or rhythmic in their body movements, but jerky, stiff and limited. The muscles of the face, shoulders and back are particularly tense.

Watch yourself, honestly, perhaps at the wheel of your car in the morning rush hour, when you're late for work. Whenever a horn sounds or a car gets in your way you can feel the muscles of your shoulders go tense. The irritations go on all day, and every time you are irritated your muscles become tense.

Then there are irritations from within you; just thinking about them can make your muscles tense: you don't like your job, you are not getting on with people, a close relative is ill, you have devastating sexual problems, and so on.

Freeing your body from tension, from restriction, from wasting its energy, is an introduction to a new world. As you start reading this book you may discover that you have never really known your body; that all your life it has been a stranger to you. But as you continue and come to know and possess your body through the book's muscle-relaxing techniques, you will come alive as perhaps never before.

# 2 Possessing your body and proprioception

## Getting to know your body

However much information you may collect *about* your body, you may still not know it – not know how to use it properly, not know how to enjoy it fully, not know how to possess it. And if you do not possess your body you are its prisoner, even though you may not be aware of it. Try a few simple tests and find out.

You bend down to touch your toes with your knees straight and find that you cannot. You raise both arms above your head and realize that you cannot reach the vertical without arching your back. You turn your head to the right as much as you can and find you cannot turn the full 90 degrees, but only 75 degrees.

Your joints are designed to make these simple movements, yet you cannot make them. You are a prisoner of your own muscles. They override your will with a will of their own which says, 'I won't'. This is then translated by you into 'I can't', and accepted as natural.

### Are you only half-alive?
You could go for a medical check-up in any Western country and be passed A1 fit without anyone fully checking how well you can move your joints. You could be passed fit but still always feel tired and without energy. Yet statistics show that rheumatic disturbance – pain located in muscles, tendons, bones and joints – is the second most widespread cause of suffering (the first is mental disturbance).

So long as you can get to work every day, put in the right number of hours, come home, enjoy your leisure, eat, drink, watch television and sleep, you may feel you are healthy and that things are going as well as can be expected. But do we just want to keep working, doing our daily tasks, with the back-up of a great medical technology that repairs us when things go wrong? It is up to us to decide first that escape from this kind of half-life is possible. This book suggests that escape is open to all and step by step will show the way.

### Moving to a fuller life
Life is movement and sensation; you are only fully alive if your body allows you full freedom of movement and full enjoyment of sensations.

Movements fall into three groups:

**1** Involuntary – which includes your internal rhythms, such as blood circulation, action of the liver and so on.
**2** Voluntary – movements governed by your will, the most obvious being movements at the joints, which are governed by your muscles.
**3** Movements that are both involuntary and voluntary, like breathing and swallowing.

It is the voluntary movements that you can improve. They are within your influence and most accessible to change.

Sensations, too, fall into different categories. Your external sense receptors (exteroceptors) are stimulated by events outside your body, producing the sensations of sight, sound, smell, taste and the sensations on the surface of your skin. Your internal sense receptors (interoceptors) are stimulated by changes inside your body, and produce feelings such as fatigue, nausea, hunger, thirst, wanting to urinate, and so on. These two types of sensation are obvious to everyone; but there is another sense, known as proprioception, and because its importance is too often ignored, let us consider it in some detail.

## What is proprioception?

How are you aware that you are standing, sitting, lying, walking, bending, lifting up your head, and so on? What is behind your body's stability, orientation, movement in space? How do you manage to stay erect and not fall over? How do you know the actions, activities and doings of your body?

The simple answer is that you have a sense for all this – the sense of your very awareness of your physical self. This is what is called proprioception; so generally neglected is this sense that there is no common or garden name for it such as all the other senses have.

Whereas exteroceptors are stimulated by external and interoceptors by internal events, proprioceptors are stimulated by both. Situated in the non-hearing part of your inner ear and in your muscles, tendons and joints, they are stimulated by the activity of your muscles, the movements of your joints, and the position of your body and its various parts. The eyes are often compared to a camera, and the ears to a microphone; in the same way, proprioception can be compared to a carpenter's spirit level. In your inner ears, muscles, tendons and joints are a complex network of tiny 'spirit levels' giving you your sense of balance, weight, position and movement.

Proprioception is your most basic sense of connection to the earth, involving your body's relationship with gravity, space and the atmosphere. It is always there in the background. While you are reading this your eyes and thinking process are active in the foreground. Yet in the background your proprioceptive sense is active, making you aware of your body – of its breathing, for instance, and its position in space.

### The most vital sense

Even loss of sight or hearing is not as devastating as loss of proprioception. Without it you would lose postural sense of your limbs and be unable to tell how they were placed without looking at them; in the dark you would lose your balance. Even though this sense may not often be totally lost it is often impaired by neglect. It cannot operate to the full in a stiff, inflexible body, but a flexible body maintains a keen sense of proprioception.

For example, by developing the fullest movements possible at your shoulder joints, you will regain sensation in the muscles which connect your shoulders to your chest. Your chest will come alive. You will feel it from the inside, that is, proprioceptively. There is a difference between knowing that, obviously, you have a chest and feeling your chest through the sensations coming from muscles, tendons and joints.

Of all your senses proprioception is the one most under your influence, through the fullest employment of your muscles. No recourse to a doctor, psychiatrist or any other outside help is needed for this. It is entirely up to you.

Being able to make the fullest use of your muscles, and therefore ensuring that the body can carry out all the movements of which it is capable, is basically a question of training your muscles to lengthen and contract as far as they were designed to.

### Battle of wills

Consider your relationship with your muscles. Simply moving your hand to your face involves the will to do it and the action of your muscles. Muscles move bones at their joints and the action happens. However, the link between will and muscle action is a mystery. Immanuel Kant said: 'That my will moves my arm is to me no more comprehensible than if someone should say that it could hold back the moon itself.'

Slowly bring your hand to your face. You have willed it and it happens. The movement is voluntary, but what muscles are used actively and passively and in what sequence and timing is an entirely automatic and unconscious matter. You have no choice, for your will directs the movements of the bones and not of the muscles themselves.

*Try this:* With your arm raised to the horizontal in front of you, first let your forearm rise to a right angle. Then bring it towards you to meet your upper arm. In the first part of the movement your biceps do the work of pulling your forearm up. But in the second part your triceps do the work of letting your forearm come to you. You make a simple voluntary movement, but you are not in the least conscious of this delicately timed co-ordination of muscle action. One group of muscles is thrown into action and the other out of action as the plumbline is crossed. It is the movement of bones by your will that is voluntary and not the muscle actions that produce the voluntary movement.

So we see that there are two aspects of every conscious action. One is the mechanical action of muscles, bones, joints and so on. The other is inner decision and judgement, the will. This continual play of muscle action and will is mostly unconscious. Every willed action or movement depends on the co-operation of muscle action. So that the more efficient the action of muscles the more effective is the operation of will.

But sometimes there appears to be a conflict between will and muscle action, as you will have realized earlier in the chapter if you couldn't touch your toes. You will a movement but your muscles do not let you carry it out. A muscle is then making you do its will, and so reducing the power of your will. You want a body immediately responsive to your will and able to function at its utmost effectiveness. This is a source of satisfaction which few other pleasures give.

**Growing in grace**
By achieving control over the muscles and hence the movements of your body you may reap many benefits:

Aches and pains caused by tension will disappear. Breathing and the circulation of the blood are improved. Supple joints add beauty to your body.

Your joints determine your posture because they bear the weight of your body as well as being the source of movement. Creating movement at every joint will automatically improve the way you hold and support your body, bringing to it a feeling of lightness and grace.

Though you cannot make yourself taller or shorter, rounded shoulders or a drooping belly can be changed. The muscles which move a particular joint are changed in shape when that joint can make all the extreme movements it is designed to make. The shape of your legs, for example, changes noticeably for the better when your hip, knee and ankle joints are flexible. If all the joints in your hands are assisted to become fully flexible, their shape changes. The most profound change can be in the area of the neck, shoulders and chest, making a vast difference to your build within the limits of the physique you were born with.

Your physical build and ability to move are probably more important in your evaluation of yourself than anything else – much more than you care to admit. Difficulty in movement undermines and distorts self-confidence. Suppleness of joints inspires self-confidence by increasing the efficiency and aliveness of your body.

### New world discovered

What we are suggesting is not merely a set of exercises that will do you good, but something more fundamental: we suggest that you can help yourself to make all the joints in your body flexible and their appropriate muscle actions efficient; that nature has designed your joints to make certain natural movements and if your joints are unable to produce them then your body is out of harmony with nature; that to promote movement is to promote sensation; that stiffness is deadness; that the life or aliveness of your body *is* its movements and sensations of itself; that it is possible to improve your posture, appearance, flexibility and strength through simple movement techniques, many of which have been practised for centuries – for instance, in gymnastics or in the Hatha Yoga tradition.

They are quite harmless and not violent. When they become too much for you, you stop. You need no training or specialization and no equipment. They cost nothing but time and attention.

As a result of these exercises your movements, sensations and body will be different. Your character will be different too, because with a different body you will have moved into a different world.

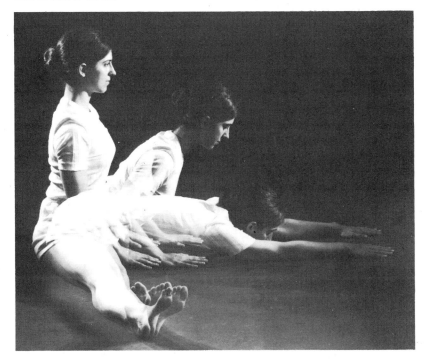

# 3 Making friends with your pain

We all hate pain. The world, we believe, would be a far better place if there were no such thing as pain. Not so. Pain is not always an evil thing that has to be punished by being ignored or driven away by drugs. More often than not we are in pain because we need to be in pain.

In the first place pain is a vital protective mechanism. People who have no pain receptors in their skin – and there are such people – cannot protect themselves from danger. They severely burn themselves, gravely injure their heads and limbs, because they do not get the early warning signal of pain.

Some pain is caused by disease or injury; this is organic pain, the pain which sends you to the doctor who can deal with it through medicines or surgery. But there is also functional pain, and this kind of pain doctors find a more difficult problem. In fact, the responsibility for handling it is our own.

One of the most obvious causes of functional pain is the overworking of your muscles. They are either contracted too long or overstretched. Most lower back pains, headaches and stiff necks are not organic but functional pains.

Let us follow through a simple example of the working of functional pain. Push your lower jaw as far forward as possible in front of your upper jaw. Now hold this until you feel the pain of overworked muscles.

**Suffering through lack of pain**
What happens if you hold your jaw forward for a day, week or month, and so on? After a time the pain will disappear, even though the pain-causing position remains. Your body will have successfully cut off the pain, because if nerve receptors are continuously overstimulated they send reduced numbers of impulses to your brain. Eventually you do not feel pain, but the price you have paid is that your jaw is now restricted in its natural movements and has also lost the normal sensations of proprioception.

In one sense it is a good thing that our bodies can adapt to pain and get on with living, otherwise we might be overwhelmed by sensations. But one's body can over-adapt to the point of danger. We have all seen people with crooked, bent bodies, shoulders rounded, hips tilted forward, whose movements are slow and awkward, who give every appearance of suffering. Yet they may feel little pain because they have restricted their movements in order not to induce it. A restricted body is, in fact, one that is in pain but without any sensation of it.

Moreover, a restricted body is very vulnerable to injury and misuse. Sensation in it is minimal. It has no guide, no protection, and suddenly, bending or twisting or lifting something, it is too late. Muscles go into acute spasm and the body cannot move for the pain.

Why should twisting, turning, bending be injurious to a body once well-designed to take these functions in its stride? The obvious answer is that not enough time and attention have been given to keeping your joints flexible. Otherwise this would never have happened. If you take the attitude that all aches and pains are the concern of doctors, then minor aches and pains, which are mostly functional, will not be attended to until they add up enough to warrant medical care. And once in this state there is not much else you can do.

To take functional pain into your own hands is best done, not when you are in intense pain and overwhelmed, but with your day-to-day aches and pains. These everyday minor ailments are the challenge.

### Be prepared for pain
To recreate a flexible body will involve discomfort and pain. You must accept that from the start. To see why let us return to the protruding jaw. If you began to bring it back into its natural position, the previous process would go into reverse and you would begin to experience the pain that had been cut off. In disturbing a bad habit and bringing back movement and sensation to your jaw some pain would be inevitable.

The problem is that most of us would rather flee from pain than face it, even at the cost of giving up intense aliveness. We would sooner turn to pain-killers, thinking that to have deadened it fastest is to have cured it best. In fact, pain-killers keep you further away from ever correcting faults of posture and bad muscle habits.

It is therefore sensible to accept those kinds of pain, discomfort or tension which are necessary and beneficial while avoiding pain which is unnecessary and harmful. Pain that comes from lengthening (i.e. relaxing) tight hamstrings or pectoral muscles, for example, is beneficial. You are disturbing a bad habit. On the other hand, pain that comes from overbending your lower back is caused by disturbing a part not designed for such an activity and is harmful.

### Beneficial and harmful pain
Harmful pain arises when active groups of muscles are overworked through over-use or when they resist a load that is too great for them. This pain is a warning signal to stop.

Beneficial pain, on the other hand, is caused when a passive muscle group, which means one that is extended to its maximum, is further lengthened. You always feel better after beneficial pain. The lengthening seems to relax the muscle group so that its relationship with its opposite is improved and when it is called upon to be active its power and efficiency is increased. It is this lengthening and relaxing of muscle action that slowly restores a proper relationship between active and passive groups of muscles at every joint, and brings flexibility back to your body.

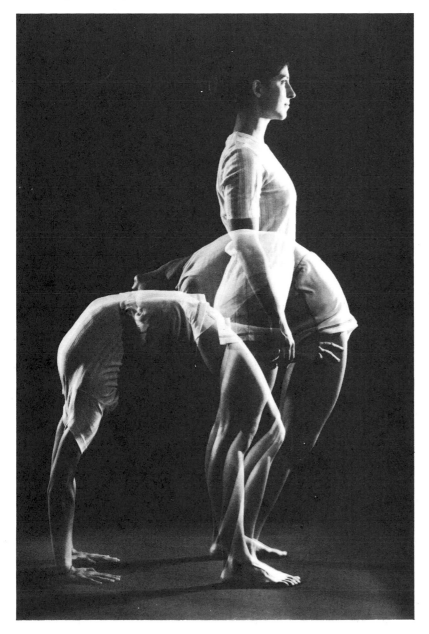

# 4 Knowing your body through touch

## *The magic in your hands*

You probably know your body most of all through looking at it. But you can add to that knowledge through your sense of proprioception and your sense of touch. The tools for learning about your body through touch are those remarkable instruments, your hands, especially since they are fitted with opposable thumbs, absent in all other animals.

Hands are also a vital tool in our programme of self-help, for massage is an ancient method of healing. It has been used in different forms for thousands of years. The word comes from the Portuguese *amassár,* to knead, but as well as kneading massage involves stroking and friction. It assists circulation and increases the suppleness of your tissues. Apart from oils and ointments it is the only way directly to treat your skin (all sixteen to twenty square feet of it).

The appearance of your skin is of enormous importance in the impression you make on others; there is no magician's mantle to compare with it. It combines the qualities of overcoat, waterproof, sunshade, suit of armour and refrigerator. It is sensitive to heat and cold, pain and the touch of a feather. It can withstand the wear and tear of seventy years and more, and it carries out its own running repairs.

### Self-discovery

There is no mystery in massage, but those who try it will be surprised at the magic they hold in their hands. The advantage of self-massage over being massaged by another person is that, as well as the gain in stimulation and well-being, you learn about your body through your hands. This is a far richer way of discovering your skeleton, joints and muscles than through a diagram.

Another person will be able to get to some parts more easily than you can and the technique used may be more professional and efficient. Yet you can, with curiosity, practice and patience, learn to reach all parts of your body and develop your own natural ways of massage. Almost instinctively you will find how to do this and you will have the advantage of being able to regulate the pressure you exert to what you can bear.

Massage, of course, especially deep massage, provokes pain. The reaction varies in different people and in different parts of your body. Indeed your body may be loaded with painful spots you are never aware of until you try massage. Mongolian warriors equated unnecessarily painful spots with fear and before and after battle they would massage their entire bodies in order to rid themselves of pain and, hence, fear.

It is indeed possible to massage painful spots away. *Try this:* Massage one of your feet, say the left, for ten minutes a day for a week. Then compare the reactions of your left foot and your right foot to various degrees of pressure. You will be astounded at the difference.

In self-massage you can use one or both hands, and any part of the hand, fingers, thumb, flat, back or sides, provided you exert enough pressure. Pressure on the skin empties the blood vessels and its release allows them to fill again, thus producing a pump action. Where possible massage in the direction of your venous flow, that is, towards your heart.

### Massage made simple

The many textbook movements of massage can be reduced to four:

1 **Surface stroking** with the flat of your hand. In severe pain or spasm it is often the only form of massage.
2 **Deep stroking,** which is done in the same way, but with greater pressure.
3 **Friction,** which is carried out by pressing with the tips of your fingers and thumbs.
4 **Kneading,** which is done by alternately squeezing and releasing a muscle.

However, an even simpler general instruction would be to explore and press, probe to find the painful parts and apply friction to dissolve the pain.

Now for a programme of massage that will allow you to get thoroughly acquainted with your body and refresh it at the same time. Take a different part of your body each week. For instance, begin with your feet, which have many joints and muscles, then go from your ankles to your knees, next from your knees to your groin, and so on.

For the less accessible parts different positions are necessary.

Your upper back between your shoulderblades is the most difficult to reach. Kneel on the floor with your forehead resting on two cushions. This position enables you to reach this area.

For your lower thoracic back lie on your side, with your head on a cushion, and use the back of your opposite hand.

A good position for massaging your neck is sitting with your head forward, supported by cushions, on a table.

The best position for massaging your abdominal muscles is lying on your back with your head on a cushion and your knees bent.

You may, of course, find other positions which suit you better.

Having massaged each section of your body week by week you should then be able to deal with your entire body in fifteen minutes. Doing this each morning gives your body the attention and invigoration it deserves and helps to prevent pain.

The only part of your body for which more detailed instructions are needed is your face, that moving panorama of muscle action.

The muscles of your face are numerous and varied, and run in every direction – in nearly straight lines, obliquely, transversely and in circles. Your face is a storehouse of muscle arrangements. This is not surprising when you consider the power of movement and expression it exhibits. In no part of your body are the muscles more numerous and complicated. Each part has its own particular muscles – your ears, eyes, nose, cheeks, chin and jaws. These muscles act singly and in combinations.

The muscles of expression can make a plain face beautiful, and can change a fine face into that of a fiend. They are mind muscles par excellence; to the ancients the face was the mirror of the mind, and no other part of the body is as expressive of emotion.

*Magic mirror on the wall,*
*Which is the tightest muscle of them all?*

Sit in front of a mirror; only this way can you see what is going on in your face. Following the diagram, locate the muscles of your head. Now try these movements:

*Raise your eyebrows in surprise.* To do that you have contracted the frontal portion of the occipito-frontalis muscle, which lies in and above your forehead. The auricularis muscle also moves in eyebrow raising.

*Move your scalp backwards and forwards.* Both front and back occipito-frontalis muscles are moving alternately.

*Wrinkle the bridge of your nose.* That is the procerus muscle at work.

*Put a finger between your eyebrows and frown.* You will feel both occipito-frontalis and procerus muscles contract.

By now you will be aware how forceful these muscle actions can be. In spite of its flexibility, your skin is a tough, thick hide. Hard and strained action is needed to crease it and keep it creased for any length of time.

*Frown as you press your temples at the edge of your eyebrows, then along your eyebrows to the bridge of your nose.* What you feel contracting is the large oval muscle that surrounds each eye, the orbicularis oculi, which extends to your eyebrow region, your temple, cheek and nose. Its main function is to close your eye forcibly, but part of it is also involved in

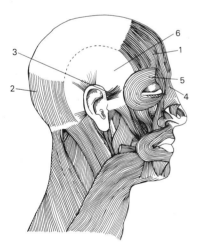

Muscles of the face, scalp and neck:
1 Front occipito-frontalis
2 Back occipito-frontalis
3 Auricularis
4 Procerus
5 Orbicularis oculi
6 Temporalis under temporal fascia

frowning. Its central portion is in your eyelids, enabling them to close gently in sleep, or snap shut as a protection against impending eye injury.

*Squint and blink your eyes forcibly several times.* Note both the contraction and hard rigidity of the tensed muscles, especially around your eye sockets and in your upper cheeks.

*Place your fingertips directly above your ears and bite down with your teeth several times, moving your fingers forward about a half-inch with each bite.* You can instantly feel the strength of the temporalis muscle, which overlies each temple. It is a biting, chewing and clenching muscle, and as such most powerful.

## Face and head massage

After you have become familiar with the muscles of your face in the mirror, try this.

Sit down and massage your forehead, temples, eyes, nose, upper jaw, lower jaw, throat, ears, scalp, back of your head and neck.

Place your fingers at the centre of *your forehead.* Now press gently, drawing your fingers outward in either direction until you reach your temples (**1**). Repeat this a few times until your entire forehead has been massaged.

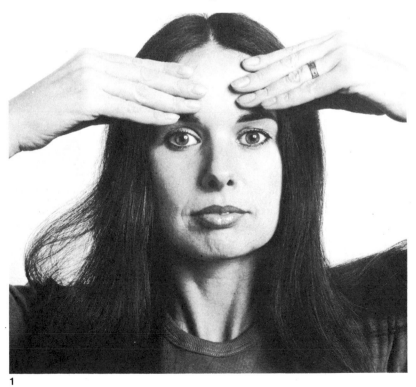

1

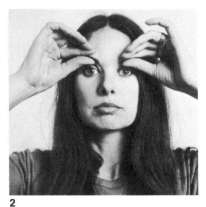

2

Pinch and pull the fleshy parts of *your eyebrows*, beginning at the bridge of your nose and working to the outer corners of your eyes (**2**).

Place the flat of your thumbs in the corners of *your eyes* under your eyebrow bones and slide gently to the outsides of your eyes (**3**). Now place your index fingers on the bony rim under your eyes and with gentle pressure slide your fingers to the outsides of your eyes (**4,5**). Close your eyes and place your index and middle fingers at the inner corners of your eyes; then gently draw them outwards across your eyes (**6**). Do these three eye massages several times.

With your thumb and index finger squeeze *your nasal bone*

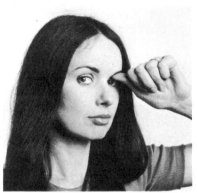

3

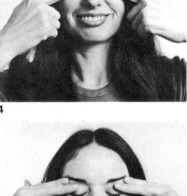

4

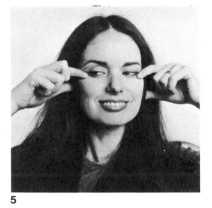

5

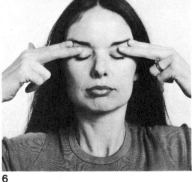

6

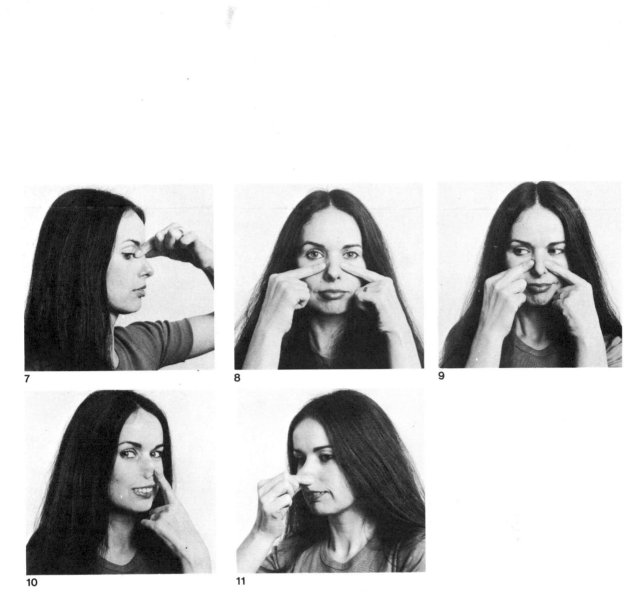

7

8

9

10

11

and press in the inner corners of your eyes (**7**). Place your index fingers on the sides of your nasal bone and massage it by gentle pressure and small circular movements (**8,9**).

With your finger bend your nose tip to the left and right (**10**), and then with thumb and index finger push to the sides and rotate the cartilage of *your nose* (**11**).

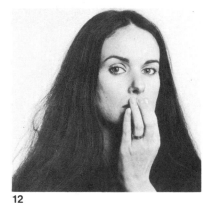

12

Use your fingers to press *the area between your nose and mouth;* start in the centre and work your top jaw as if you were massaging your upper gums from the outside (**12**).

Place the tips of your forefingers and middle fingers alongside your nose, just below the lower rims of your eye sockets (**13**). Pressing firmly but gently, trace a path across *your cheeks* to *your temples,* then along your lower cheeks to your temples (**14**). With your fingers resting on your head, use your thumbs to massage your temples in a series of small circles (**15, 16**). Finally, press your thumbs into the base of your cheekbones and hold for thirty seconds (**17**).

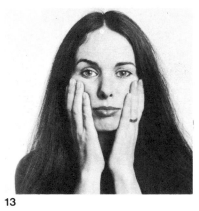

13

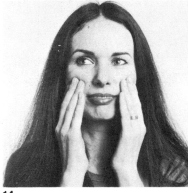

14

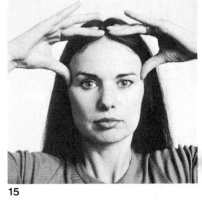

15

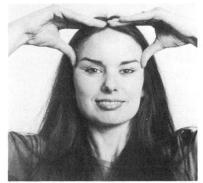

16

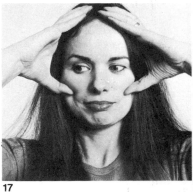

17

26

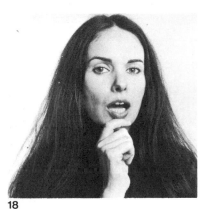

**18**

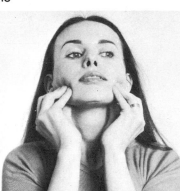

**19**

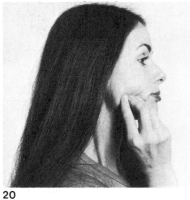

**20**

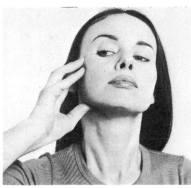

**21**

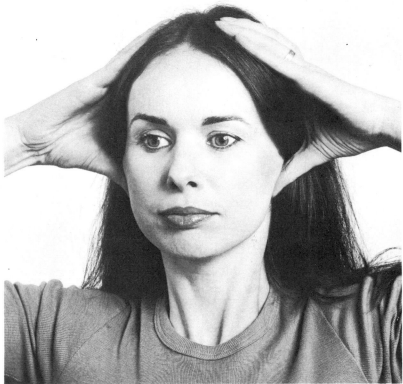

**22**

With your index finger and thumb, 'milk' *your chin* above and below (**18**). Then with your fingers on top and your thumbs below press and trace a path from the centre of your chin to the ends of your lower jawbones just below your ears (**19, 20**). Where your jawbones curve upwards, press the bone and hold for fifteen seconds (**21**). Finally, with your fingers on your head and your thumbs on the sides of your jawbones, massage using small circular movements (**22**).

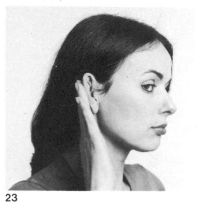

**23**

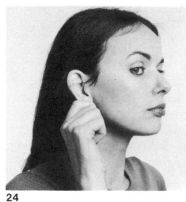

**24**

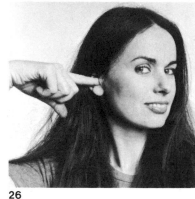

**25**

**26**

Flip *your ears* forward, flatten them hard against the sides of your head, brush them forward repeatedly (**23**). Pull your earlobes down a few times (**24**). Now, with a finger trace the spiral of each ear (**25**). Use the tip of your finger to rub all around the spiral channel of your ear. Start at the top and end in the ear proper (**26**).

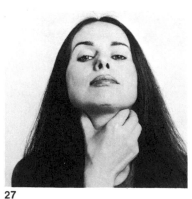

**27**

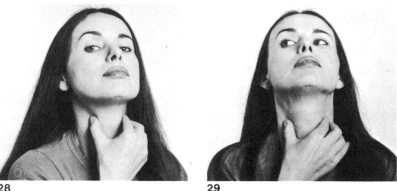

**28**

**29**

Place your finger and thumb on *your hyoid bone* at the top of your throat; gently swing it from left to right (**27**). Do the same with *your voice box* (**28**). Now, make long strokes from the top of your throat to its base (**29**). Repeat several times.

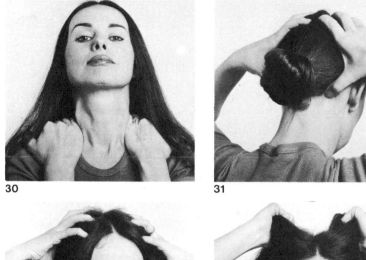

30

31

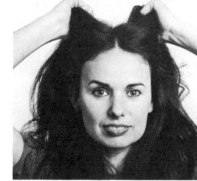

32

33

With your hands grip the muscles connecting *your neck* to your shoulders (**30**). Tighten and release several times. Place your hands behind your neck, pressing gently with all your fingers in the area on either side of your spine. Begin as far down your back as you can. Then, wriggling or circling your fingertips as you press, move your fingers up to the base of your skull. Now press with both thumbs into the base of your skull (**31**). Work the base of your skull thoroughly.

Place all your fingers and thumbs on your head, moving *your forehead and scalp* as you massage quite forcibly (**32**). Finally, grasp handfuls of *hair* and pull up, around and back and forth until your scalp tingles (**33**).

This face and head self-massage can be done any time you find convenient, but a good time is first thing in the morning. It is also very helpful when you have a headache.

Getting acquainted with your face through massage in the mirror teaches you to become aware of its muscles so that you begin to sense what they are doing throughout the day. You will soon begin catching yourself as you unwittingly frown, clench your teeth, set your jaw, thrust your head forward and so on. Once caught, such expressions can be exchanged for others that do not bring tension.

# 5 Bones

### Your lively skeleton

Your skeleton is made up of 206 bones, so linked together that your body can stand, sit, walk, run, jump and bend in a great variety of ways. Some bones are long, like your arm and leg bones, your ribs and collarbones. Some are flat, like those of your skull and hips, your breastbone and shoulderblades. Other bones are irregular, such as, for example, those making up your backbone, your wrists and the weight-bearing parts of your feet.

Your skeleton has three principal mechanical functions – support, movement and protection.

### The supporting skeleton

Like a system of internal girders, the skeleton supports and maintains your body shape. Improve the way your skeleton supports your body and you improve the appearance of your body.

The mechanical, supporting function of your skeleton is to bear the weight of your body masses as it passes downward from your head to your trunk, to your pelvis, and legs and through your feet to the ground, whether you are at rest or moving. Your weight is carried through a flexible column of jointed parts (backbone) and is transferred through a rocking base (pelvis) to two jointed supports (legs), resting on the ground. If the line of thrust is centred through your joints, your posture will be balanced and your muscle actions efficient. You will use your energy economically. If the thrust is not centred there will be unequal pulls on muscles and adjoining tissues, causing stress, strain and pain, using up and wasting much energy and effort.

### The moving skeleton

Bones act as levers in movement and joints are the source of movement. Skeleton and muscles together make movement possible.

Anatomists think of the skeleton in two parts. One is the axial skeleton, which includes skull, backbone, breastbone and ribs and is the axis of your body. The second part is the appendicular skeleton, made up of pelvis and shoulder girdles, legs and arms – appendages to the axis. If you allow your shoulders, arms, legs and pelvis (the appendicular skeleton) to become stiff and limited you will force your axial skeleton to

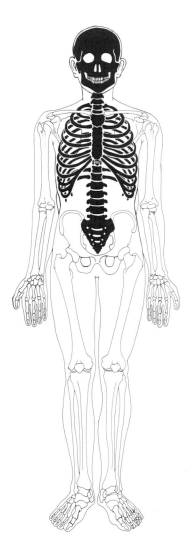

Axial skeleton in solid, appendicular skeleton in outline

work unnecessarily in most of the movements you make. The way to overcome this misuse and over-use of your body is to make your shoulders, arms, legs and pelvis flexible.

**Your protective skeleton**

The architecture of your skeleton protects delicate parts. Your skull encases your brain and your backbone encases your spinal cord. Your ribcage encloses your heart and lungs, yet is flexible enough to expand and contract with every breath.

Now let us take a closer look at the positions and roles of the major bones in the body and their relationship with one another, before turning to the joints and muscles which bring bones into movement.

**Well-balanced head**

Your skull is the skeleton of your head and face. It is made up of twenty-one bones, immovably bound together in joints called sutures. Your head, which weighs about 15 to 20 lb (7 to 9 Kg), sits and balances on the neck part of your backbone at the point just behind your ears where your jaws articulate and in line with the entrance to your ears. It is not hanging from a hinge joint at the back of your neck.

*Try this:* Start your head nodding gently, like a toy mandarin, keeping your eyes focused on one point, and you will at once sense where your head rests on your neck.

**Plenty of backbone**

Many people seem to think of their backbone as the bumps they can feel just under the skin in their back. In fact, your backbone is deep-set, occupying about half the diameter of your body from front to back.

It is a jointed column made up of twenty-six vertebrae (from the Latin *vertere* – to turn), which fall into five groups:

**1** Seven cervical vertebrae, the same number as in a mouse or giraffe, compose your neck, hold up your head and indirectly support your top chest, shoulders and arms.
**2** Twelve thoracic vertebrae, plus your ribs and breastbone, form your chest.
**3** Five lumbar (lower back) vertebrae, the largest and deepest vertebrae, complete the flexible part of your backbone. They are the vertebrae of your loins, in ancient times regarded as the centre of strength and generative powers.
**4** Five sacral vertebrae fuse into a shield-shaped plate called the sacrum, the largest part of the backbone, which bears the accumulated weight of head, shoulders, arms and trunk and leans on the two hip bones.
**5** Four or five vertebrae fused together make up your coccyx, perhaps the remnant of a tail.

Man, unlike most other animals, walks upright. The result is that his backbone has a load-bearing function which it does not have in animals that go on all fours. To adapt to this, curves are necessary, and the structure of the backbone ensures that it is not straight but S-shaped, arranged like a snake in four opposing curves. These curves enable it to support weights that are not directly in line with the centre of gravity. (When you talk about keeping your back straight, that does not mean straightening it out like a board but only keeping its curvature at a minimum.)

### The yoke you carry

Your shoulder girdles (that is, your collarbones and shoulderblades) hang from your head and neck and their weight is carried by your backbone. They are a yoke-like arrangement hung across the top of your chest, not connected directly to your backbone at any point. The only bony connection is through your collarbones to your breastbone, which in turn is connected to your backbone by your ribs. Thus your shoulder girdles hang quite free of your chest, your collarbones acting like yardarms to keep your shoulders free from your chest. (If your collarbone is snapped your shoulder collapses on to your chest.)

Your shoulder girdles serve to anchor your arms, which fit into them at your shoulder joints and hang from them. Your triangular, shield-shaped shoulderblades hang at the sides of your chest and not at the back of it as many people imagine.

The whole design is such as to enable your arms to move freely and powerfully without bringing any pressure on the upper part of your chest where your heart and lungs are.

### An airy cage

Your chest is a strong, egg-shaped cage, often called your ribcage. The first two pairs of ribs and the top part of your breastbone hang mainly by muscles connected to your head and neck. All the rest hang from the thoracic vertebrae – thus your chest exerts a side load on your backbone from your head to the last thoracic vertebra.

The dimensions of your chest change rhythmically about eighteen to twenty times a minute with the movements of breathing. Each rib has its own range and direction of movement contributing to the combined breathing movement.

The chest's supporting role is important. Your ribs and breastbone provide strong, widespread attachments for the stretchable parts of your trunk – that is, muscles, tendons, ligaments and adjoining tissues. This makes up the great muscle and tendon-like wall of the front of your body. Your chest is so made that its weight and movements are balanced in relation to those of the upper and lower portions of your body.

The total action of these stretchable tissues produces a force equal to that of the compressing bones of your back.

## Arm's length

There are sixty bones in your upper limbs, and of these fifty-four are in your hands. Each upper arm contains a single bone, jointed to your shoulderblade. Two bones run through your forearm and when you hold out your hands, palms upwards, they lie side by side parallel along their entire length. When you turn your palm downwards, the one bone (the radius) crosses over the other (the ulna) just above your wrist.

## Hips to toes

The skeleton of the lower limbs includes your hip bones, thighs, leg and feet bones. The hip bones (see diagram) are:

**1** The ilia, which is the bony rim that can be felt going around half your body – the part on which you rest your hands on your hips.
**2** The ischia or buttock bones, on which your body rests when sitting.
**3** The pubes, the bones of your groin above your genitals.

These hip bones, plus your sacrum and coccyx, which belong to your backbone, are together called the pelvis. The pelvis sits on your thigh bones. The weight of your entire trunk is transferred from your pelvis to your thighs at your hip joints, then to your knees and from your knees via your shin bones to your ankles. The weight from your ankle bones is then distributed at right angles to the twenty-five bones of each foot in a series of arches.

## Blood and bone bank

Your skeleton has two other uses. Bone marrow supplies your body with red blood cells – 200,000 million a day – some white blood cells and platelets. Red blood cells carry oxygen. White cells ingest invading germs, and platelets allow clotting to stop accidental bleeding. Your bones are also your body's mineral bank, storing calcium carbonate and calcium phosphate.

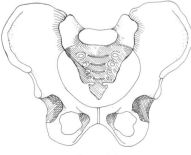

The pelvis

# 6 Joints

## *The why and how of movement*

Bones could not move without joints, and muscles are needed to bring joints into action. This chapter concentrates on the body's hundred and one joints, but must begin with the caution that even though you consider its parts separately the body works only as a whole and depends on the co-ordinated power of every part.

Joints are the places where bones meet bones. In your skeleton they are the source of movement, the points where weights are transferred, the source of proprioceptive sensation and the centre of relationship between one part of the body and its adjoining and all other parts.

**The joint for the job**

The construction of a joint depends on the job it has to do. If a joint is round in all directions, like the ball-and-socket joints of your shoulders and hips, it permits a great deal of movement. If it is a simple hinge joint, like your elbows, the movements are limited to bending and extending.

The linings of movable joints are of two kinds. In some joints, the tissue between the bones is cartilage. The cartilage that separates the bones of your backbone is in the form of discs which act as buffers. They allow your backbone to move, bend and extend while at the same time protecting it from undue stress. In the centre of each disc is a fluid mass which enables it to act as a shock absorber. The more movable the section of your backbone, the larger the discs. Thus, in your neck, the discs make up about 40 per cent of its length, in your lumbar region, 33 per cent, and in your thoracic region, only about 20 per cent. Excess strain on your backbone from supporting unbalanced weights and from over-use and misuse can make the discs protrude from the joints. Such discs are commonly described as 'slipped'.

Very few of the joints in your limbs have a lining of tissue. Instead there is a cavity containing a lubricating fluid called synovial fluid. The ends of the bones are covered with cartilage, a smooth, glossy substance that reduces friction to a minimum.

Synovial joints may be plane, hinge, saddle, pivot, ball-and-socket or cone shaped. The movements they can make are:

**1 Gliding,** which occurs in every synovial joint as a simple movement of one surface over another.

**2 Angular,** as at a hinge joint like your elbow. *Try this:* Bend your arm; this is 'flexion'. Straighten your elbow; this is 'extension'. At ball-and-socket shoulder and hip joints, angular movements of arm or leg can be made in four directions. As well as forward (flexion) and backward (extension) movements, outward and inward movements are also possible. The outward movement, away from your body, is 'abduction', the movement in towards your body, 'adduction'.

**3 Rotating,** which is the movement of a bone around its own axis. *Try this:* Hold your arm extended and turn your palm alternately face up and face down. You can feel the upper arm bone, the humerus, rotating on its own axis.

**4 Circular** (or circumductive), which means the joint allows a circular movement. This is the freest and largest kind of movement.

## Universal joints

You can also have combinations of all four movements, giving 'universal' movement. Head, trunk, legs and arms can all be said to have universal movement.

At the upper end of your backbone is a joint on which your head can be made to turn to the right or left, to the extent of nearly a quarter of a turn. Your trunk can be made to turn to the right or left to about the same extent. Into these turning movements a certain amount of spiralling enters.

Your trunk can bend forward or backward and also curve to the right and left sides. Your trunk, with feet on the ground as a fixed point, can be made to circumduct. The various movements can be made to run into each other. Thus the circular turning and spiralling can be combined with more or less pronounced forward and backward bending movements, in front, back or side directions, so that a universality of movement may be claimed for your trunk.

Your head in its own right and your trunk as a whole can both be said to have a universality of movement. Other universal joints are your hip joints and shoulder joints. All these movements vary according to the agility of each individual, but all can be improved in range and efficiency.

Bearing in mind the relationship between all parts of the body, we can now take a voyage of exploration of the hundred and one joints, repeating the route taken along the bones of your body in the previous chapter. As you proceed, you will get some idea of what individual joints are capable of, and whether you are using them to the utmost.

## Some neck!

The joint between your head and your first neck vertebra, which is called the atlas vertebra (Atlas was a Greek demi-god who held up the sky), allows forward and backward bending, as when you nod your head, a slight sideways tilting to either side, but no rotation. Forward and backward mobility of your head is increased by the movement of your neck. Bending to the sides is largely done by your neck as a whole and only slightly by the head joint itself. Rotation, on the other hand, occurs almost exclusively at the joint between your first and second neck vertebrae (between your atlas and axis). Thus all the movements of your head – other than rotation – are assisted by the movements of your neck as a whole.

*Try this:* Take your head forwards, let your chin touch your breastbone, then extend it backwards, lifting your chin as high as possible. Turn your head to the left and then to the right. Now place your left ear as close as possible to your shoulder, then the same with the other side. Finally, using the centre of your head as a pointer describe a circle clockwise, then anti-clockwise. It is clear that the seven vertebrae and eight joints of your neck as a unit truly make up a universal joint.

## What your backbone can and can't do

In your entire backbone there are twenty-six joints. The intervertebral discs allow the vertebrae to rock upon each other, compressing one side of each disc and expanding the opposite side. These small movements added together result in free bending of your backbone as a whole. It can flex forward, extend backward and bend sideways. In addition, the discs allow slight rotation between vertebrae.

Extension is the freest of all the backbone's movements. In fact, as can be seen on pages 19 and 113, the potential for backward bending is remarkable. It is greatest in your lumbar region, free in your neck and reduced in your thoracic region. Many people are unaware of this potential to bend their trunk backwards and stiff backs are so common as to be regarded as normal. Few doctors even consider an immobile backbone as a lack of functional health. If we can't bend backwards we think 'We are made that way' and 'It can't be helped'. If we see someone else bending their trunk backwards we conclude that they are 'double-jointed'. No one is double-jointed. There is no such thing.

Flexion, or forward bending of your trunk, is on the whole far more restricted by the design of the backbone than backward bending. Overbending and a rounded trunk are unnatural and a strain on your body. But because we spend so much of our day slouched or bent over, the muscles and tissues in front of our trunk have become short and restricting, those of the back overstretched and strained. Natural forward bending of your trunk which appears to be flexion of your backbone is in fact mostly flexion of your hip joints. Your backbone is not designed to bend too far forward. All the later exercises focus on reducing forward bending of your backbone and increasing it at your hip joints.

*Try this:* With your knees slightly flexed, bend forwards (in this movement your hip joints flex and so do all the vertebrae of your backbone). Now extend backwards as far as possible, head going back and hips forward.

Next, keeping your hips square, take your left arm down as far as it can go, side-bending your backbone. Do the same on the other side. Still keeping your hips firmly square, rotate your trunk to turn as far to the left side as possible, as if you were trying to look behind you. Do the same to the right.

Finally, with hips still firm and square, using your head as a pointer and your neck straight and firm, describe a circle with the source of the movement in your lower back or lumbar, clockwise then anti-clockwise.

From this you will realize that your backbone as a whole is another universal joint.

## Grace through shoulders

The next joints to explore are those of your shoulders. They are the freest and most used, and have the advantage of not supporting any great weight. At the same time they most easily distort your body when they are limited in movement. Because they are in constant use their full flexibility is essential to a well-balanced, supple and graceful body.

The joints where your collarbones meet your breastbone are capable of movements in many directions but the range is restricted. The joints between your collarbones and shoulderblades allow a small degree of gliding movement. The most important joints of your shoulder girdles are those between your shoulderblades and your chest. They allow movements of your shoulderblades on the side and back of your chest wall. Your shoulderblades may be depressed or elevated, as when you shrug your shoulders, protracted as in pushing, or retracted as in bringing back your shoulders, and rotated to turn your arms upwards.

*Try this:* Place your left hand on your right collarbone, spreading your fingers along the bone. Now move your right arm forwards, backwards, outwards, inwards. Note that the collarbone moves with the various arm movements. Now place your left hand on your right shoulderblade. Your palm should be on its top and your fingers under a bone called the shoulderblade's spine. Raise your arm to the vertical and feel the blade rotate outwards. Take your arm behind your back as far as possible. This time your shoulderblade rotates inwards.

From these two experiences you will see that your shoulder

joint works in co-ordination with your collarbone and shoulderblade. Your collarbones articulate with your breastbone and your shoulderblades. And your shoulderblades in turn articulate with your arm bones.

**Arms round-up**

Thanks to your shoulder joints, your arms can hang flexed at your sides, or you can extend them backwards, forwards and sideways and rotate them inwards or outwards. All these combine to allow circular movements.

To discover the kinds of movement your shoulder joints allow your arms to make, *try this:* Stand up and raise your arms to the vertical above your head. Cross them behind your head and in front of your head. Next, let them hang at your sides, then cross them in front of your chest and behind your back. Relax them at your sides and then, interlocking your fingers behind you, take them as far back as possible. Then hold your arms out extended to your sides and rotate them in the sockets of your shoulder joints, first palm down and back and then palm up and back. Finally, using your hand as a pointer, describe the largest circle you can with each arm in turn.

When your arms are raised erect forwards or sideways, there is movement throughout your shoulderblades, collarbones and arms, of their joints, ligaments and muscles. About 60 degrees of this movement is achieved through the rotation of your shoulderblades, the remaining 120 degrees through the movement of your shoulder joints. There is a variation among people in the angle through which their arms can be raised. You can easily determine this for yourself.

*Try this:* Lie on the floor with your knees tucked in and feet on a wall and buttocks touching the wall. Now, with your elbows straight, take your arms overhead as close to your ears as possible (see page 64). The angle at which your arms lie on the floor will indicate how far upwards you can extend your arms.

Another movement which is often restricted is that of backward extension of the arms.

*Try this:* Sit on your feet, bend forward and extend your arms backwards with your hands interlocked.

The amount of rotation of the arm at the shoulder joint also varies between individuals.

*Try this:* Flex your elbows at right angles and using your forearms as pointers rotate your arms outwards.

Each elbow is a simple hinge joint where your upper arm bone meets your two forearm bones and it can bend and extend only.

Examine the movements of your wrist. It can bend forward, extend backward, move slightly sideways and make circular movements clockwise and anti-clockwise.

*Try this:* Hold your arms out in front of you, palms down. Now bend your wrists, bringing your hands up and back towards you. Check whether you have the ability to bend your wrists at a perfect right angle. Now drop your hands and bend your wrists the other way. Again you should be able to bend them at a perfect right angle.

## You have to hand it to your thumbs

Take your right hand, make a fist and count all the joints that are flexed – three on each finger and two on your thumb; total, fourteen joints. Now open your hand. All fourteen joints also allow extension.

Keeping your hand open, bring your fingers together and then take them apart. From this you may conclude that all the lower joints also have sideways movement. This is the extent of voluntary movement, but if you use your right hand to assist the movements of your left hand and vice versa, you add rotating movements to the flexing, extending and sideways movements. Thus one hand helps the other to take all the movements a hand can do to their extreme limit.

Two angular movements at right angles to each other occur at your thumb, that is, to and fro and side to side. These combine to make circular movements, vital to the working of your hand.

*Try this:* Write without using your thumb. You will find that by themselves your fingers cannot do very much, but thumb and fingers together open up an enormous range of manipulations. Man's thumbs are unique – no other animal has them. Indeed, it is arguable that it is mainly thanks to his thumbs that man has become master of the world.

## Expansive chest

While your ribs move in conformity with your backbone, the essential movement of your chest is concerned with increasing and decreasing its capacity in breathing. Where your ribs join your backbone, there is a slight gliding movement and where they meet your breastbone, a slight rotation and twisting. This allows a pivoting of your ribs so that each pair can swing like a bucket handle. Your chest is capable of expansion in all directions. However, for convenience, consider it as a single movable cage, attached to the twelve thoracic vertebrae of your backbone.

## The load on your hips

Your hip bones are large and support a large weight. There are four movable joints. Two joints are located where your sacrum (the base of your backbone) is braced by your hip bones in your lower back. These have very little movement, a slight rocking forward and backward only.

The other two joints, where your thigh bones meet your hips, are large ball-and-socket, i.e. universal joints; after your knee joints these are the largest in your body and they are second only to your shoulder joints in range. They are under great strain, for they must both support the weight of your body and allow your hips to move. The bearing surfaces are so perfect a fit that any small defect may seriously impair movement and throw undue strains upon other joints, especially those of your lower back.

*Try these:*

**1** *To bring home to you that the hip joint is a universal joint and that your legs can move in all directions:* Stand on one leg supporting yourself against a table or a wall. Now swing the free leg forward, backward, sideways, away from your other leg, inwards in front of your other leg and behind it. Rotate your entire limb inwards and outwards. Finally, describe a circle with your foot as a pointer.

**2** *To flex your hip joints to their extreme limit:* Stand with knees straight; allow your trunk to descend as far as possible, as if you were touching your toes. Or, sitting on your heels, bend forward, taking your belly to your thighs. (This flexion is easier because your knees are flexed.)

**3** *To extend your hip joints to their maximum:* Sit between your feet and slowly lie down on your back (see page 106).

**4** *To open your legs fully:* Lie on the floor, buttocks against a wall with legs on the wall forming a wide 'V' angle. Let your legs open as wide as possible (see page 96).

**5** *To rotate your thigh bones to their maximum:* Sit between your feet to bring them inwards (see page 100) and then sit in the tailor position (see page 92) to bring them outwards.

## Big knees, simple ankles, versatile feet

Your knees are your largest joints and their movements are flexion, extension and slight rotation inwards and outwards. In full extension, produced mainly by your front thigh muscles, all the ligaments are taut, so that the joints are said to be locked.

When your legs are not bearing weight, especially if your knees are half flexed, there is a small degree of rotation, inwards and outwards, of your shin bones against your thigh bones. This outward rotation of your shin bones, plus the outward rotation of your thigh bones at your hip joints, allows you – with practice – eventually to sit in the lotus position (see page 105). Inward rotation of shin bones and thigh bones allows you to sit between your feet.

Your ankle joint is a loose hinge and the action of calf muscles can straighten out a foot so far that ballet dancers can walk on the tips of their toes with ease.

*Try this:* Move your ankles around and you will discover that they can take your feet away from your legs (plantar-flexion) and towards your legs (dorsi-flexion), and not much more. To take these two movements to their extremes, first sit on your feet, which widens the angle between your feet and your legs, and then squat on your heels, supported if need be. This position brings your feet as close as possible to your legs.

There are thirty joints in your feet and their movements are similar to those of the thirty joints in your hands — except that your big toes are nowhere near as versatile as your thumbs.

## When joints are out of joint

Your capacity for subtle and complicated movements is enormous, as this brief tour of your body has shown. While you may have found your range of movements limited at some of your joints in various ways, it is a fact that by using the proper techniques this can in time be dramatically increased.

As well as allowing movement, most joints transmit the weight of one part of your body to another. For example, at your hip joints the weight of your head, shoulders, arms and trunk is transferred to your legs. Where weight is transferred, the cartilage at the ends of the bones has to stand up to a lot of wear and tear and may become so rough that some people can feel the surfaces of their joints grating together with every movement. This common affliction is arthritis, or inflammation of the joints. Rheumatoid arthritis usually starts between the ages of twenty and forty. Older people experience another sort called osteoarthritis. Both involve a narrowing of the space between the bones in a joint which ordinarily allows them to move freely over one another.

The most susceptible joints are those which take the most strain and stress. Very often hip joints are attacked but the most common site is the backbone, which has a lifetime of stress in keeping a body upright, and is very often over-used and misused because of immobile hip and shoulder joints.

With arthritis, the entire backbone may seize up. Gradually the vertebrae have more and more difficulty in moving over one another. Some may fail completely and become totally immobile. If your hip and shoulder joints are kept flexible, it automatically follows that they support weight efficiently. You will not then over-use your backbone, and will therefore avoid unnecessary and speedy wear and tear, as well as pain.

# 7 Muscles

## *Muscle power*

When you go for a thorough medical check-up, you are given an electrocardiogram, your blood pressure and pulse rate are taken, your nervous system, eyes and ears are tested, your blood and urine are analysed, and your heart and lungs are examined. But no one examines whether your neck, back or shoulders can perform the full movements they are designed to make. Yet your muscles and the mobility of your joints have a tremendous effect on your overall health. Muscles in particular exert a great influence, for better or worse, on your metabolism and emotional life.

Your muscles do countless things for you. When you walk or move or work, you use your muscles. When you work with your hands, you use muscles. Your muscles are your means of communication with the outer world, with others: when you show your thoughts and feelings by facial movements, when you talk, write, dance, you use your muscles.

Your muscles are also the principal organs of proprioception; and they are, in a way, organs of sense, for when they go into prolonged contraction we experience pain. For instance, neglect or abuse the muscle groups that keep your body erect and you are bound to experience back pain, shoulder pain, a stiff neck or a tension headache. Muscles are also the organs of feelings such as tightness or pressure. They are instruments of perception as well as of action.

And you, and you alone, are responsible for them. They are only as good as you make them. In this area of medicine, drugs and surgery are no match for intelligent exercise and movement. No equipment, drugs or surgery are needed, no expertise or years of training or study. All you need is some simple techniques and principles and the rest is up to you.

The first step towards giving muscles the respect they deserve is to understand them. This section of the book is therefore of the utmost importance. In this and succeeding chapters we first consider what muscles are, and how they work, and look at the part they play in blood circulation. We then complete the tour of the body in which we have already explored bones and joints, to pinpoint the major muscles.

### Voluntary and involuntary
As a material, muscle does not appear very effective: when removed from the body muscles are simply lumps of meat.

Even when in full working order, muscles – which typically are ropes made of many thin fibres – can perform only one simple mechanical action, the contraction of their fibres. This means that a muscle can pull or squeeze but can never push. Yet the combination of muscles and bones in a living person produces a machine of remarkable power and delicacy.

There are two kinds of muscles, described as 'smooth' and 'striped'. *Smooth* muscles are those found in the walls of your blood vessels, guts and glands. They are not ordinarily under the control of your will and are, therefore, known as 'involuntary' muscles. *Striped* muscles are attached to your skeleton, as in your arms, legs, trunk, neck and head. These are known as 'voluntary' muscles, meaning that they are ordinarily under the control of your will. But this is not altogether so: you conceive a movement and will that it be done, but the means by which it is done are entirely automatic and beyond your control. So muscles are not voluntary, although movements are. (Your heart is a muscle whose tissues have qualities of both voluntary and involuntary muscles.)

## Tendons and ligaments

Your skeletal muscles are sheathed by fascia, which is another form of connective tissue. Most of them are attached at each end to bone, and sometimes to thick fascial bands by tendons, which are tough fibrous tissues. These save the use of long, specialized muscle fibres when short fibres are sufficient for the movement required. They also act as buffers protecting your limbs against sudden strain and acceleration.

Some muscles, although attached to bones, are inserted into your skin, such as, for example, the muscles that make a smile or frown.

Ligaments, which are made of tissue that is flexible and resistant to tension, bind your bones together but do not actually move or support them. They become taut as the bones of a joint move to their most extreme stretched position. At full stretch or in an extreme position joints are most stable, because ligaments tighten and hold them in position.

On the one hand, gradual exercise of the ligaments can stretch them positively. This is why gymnasts can perform such amazing feats and why the yogi can wrap his feet around his neck. The fingers of the Indian dancer bend backwards because constant practice has stretched the ligaments and lengthened the surrounding muscles.

On the other hand, if muscles are weak or paralysed, ligaments may overstretch from constant strain. For example, if the ligaments of the foot are stretched because of lack of muscle support, the bones of the foot may become displaced. When this happens the arch of the foot drops and one is said to be flat-footed.

## The mechanics of muscles

Every muscle is linked with the circulation by an artery and a vein. The artery brings oxygen and other essential nutrients, while the vein takes away waste products.

Muscles are allowed to use oxygen faster than your lungs and circulations can deliver it. They incur an overdraft. When an athlete pants at the end of a race he is repaying his oxygen debt. The reason is that lungs are not very good at capturing oxygen from the air. To put 1 litre of oxygen into your blood you have to take in about 20 litres of air. A 100-yarder would need 7 litres of oxygen. During the 10 seconds spent in running this distance his lungs cannot deliver more than about half a litre of oxygen to his blood. But muscles do not give up when they have used all their oxygen; they continue to work and produce lactic acid, which releases a certain amount of energy.

A muscle generates heat when it is working. That is why exercise makes you warm. Circulating blood removes surplus heat and distributes it to cooler parts or to the blood vessels near the skin, where it is lost through perspiration.

The control system regulating the timing and force of muscle contraction is represented by slender nerve fibres. At the junction of a nerve fibre and a muscle, there is a chemical amplifier. Arrival of the impulse down the nerve causes the release of a chemical (acetylcholine) which stimulates the contraction of muscle fibre. One nerve fibre serves several muscle fibres, which contract together as a single unit.

## What muscles do

Your body has more than six hundred skeletal muscles, varying in size, shape, power, speed and the ways they are connected with bones and other tissues. Each has its particular purpose. There are four classes:

**1 Prime movers,** which are the main muscles actively producing a movement. For example, when you bend your elbow, the biceps of your upper arm contract and are the prime movers.

**2 Antagonists,** which are situated in opposition to the prime movers and relax (lengthen) as the prime movers contract. Obviously, this relaxation is just as important as the contraction of the prime movers. Indeed, relaxation is the important feature in most of the positions and movements described in this book. Therapeutic gymnastics should be balanced to give both the full contraction and full relaxation of a muscle or group of them.

**3 Fixation** muscles, which steady one part, so providing a firm base for movements produced by other muscles. For example, the muscles attached to your shoulderblade steady it so that your arm may be moved at your shoulder joint.

**4 Synergists,** which act in conjunction with prime movers to help in fixing joints where movement is not wanted or to prevent an unwanted movement at the active joint.

These four classes of muscles take part in the majority of movements. A muscle does not act alone. It works in association with others, affecting movement in various ways.

*Try this:* Press your forefinger and thumb together very gently. You will find that the other fingers of the same hand are not freely mobile and that the firmer your forefinger and thumb are pressed together the stiffer the other fingers become.

Co-operative action may be taken by muscles far from the main movement. For example, movements of the eyes occur in unison with those of your head, neck and trunk. Another example: before you rise from a chair, your feet must first of all be moved backwards.

## The devil gravity

Every movement you make depends on the relationship between two opposing groups of muscles. But there is a third power that muscles have to deal with, and that is weight, or the power of gravity.

Gravity is the devil that is always pulling you down, capable of causing speedy wear and tear on your body. You have to trick the devil into aiding the power of your body, rather than dissipating and weakening it. You can never destroy gravity, but you can use it to your advantage – or not.

The force of gravity either assists or resists each movement you make. If you are standing and drop your head forward, gravity helps the movement. On the other hand, if you are lying down on your back and bend your head forward, gravity is resisting your movement.

The therapeutic positions in this book make use of the relationship between muscle action and gravity, most of them using its assistance rather than its resistance. Examples:

When you bend your body forward from your hip joints from the standing position with knees straight, you allow your trunk to be taken by gravity which stretches, lengthens and rests the hamstring muscles at the back of your thighs.

When you lie on your back with legs apart on the wall; here the weight of your lower limbs (that is, legs and thighs) surrenders to the pull of gravity. This lengthens and rests your adductor muscles on the inner sides of your thighs.

When balancing upside down, your body has the opportunity of resisting, or rather actively meeting, the forces of gravity.

### Balance building

Body building is based on the principle that strong use of a
muscle builds up muscle bulk. Body balancing – which is our
therapeutic gymnastics – is based on the principles of
lengthening and resting a muscle by outside force. The more a
muscle is stretched the greater is its capacity thereafter to
contract when needed. In this way we achieve a balance of
muscles when the prime mover and its antagonist can fully
contract and fully relax.

If all the muscles acting on a joint can, through the extreme
movements of which the joint is capable, fully relax and fully
contract, then at rest their action will be balanced.

How do you balance the action of muscles on your joints, on
your bones? Let's take ankle joints as an example. Each joint
has two extreme movements: it can be plantar-flexed or
dorsi-flexed. Now look for a way, a position, whereby, if
possible, you can make these two movements in the extreme,
using the force of your own weight to do it. Sitting between
your feet forces your lower leg (shin) bones to rotate and the
weight of your body, indirectly forcing your knees down, is
transmitted to your plantar-flexed feet. In order for this
movement to take place, the front muscles of your leg and foot,
acting on your ankles, which are the antagonists, must relax
and lengthen and the prime movers must contract sufficiently.

Now try the opposite movement. One way is to squat. With
heels flat on the ground you bend your knees and sit on your
haunches. This is a very common Eastern and African sitting
position. Another way is in the 'dog' position: hands and feet
apart, knees straight, elbows straight, heels on the ground and
body or chest angled towards your feet (see page 90). Both
these positions now demand the reverse of the sitting position
in the previous test.

The prime movers of that position now become the
antagonists, or muscles preventing the movement. The back
muscles of your shin bones are now lengthened and rested.

If these movements can be done with ease we can say that
the muscles acting on the ankle joints are in balanced action,
in that they are capable of full contraction as prime movers and
full relaxation as antagonists. Their neutral position will be in
harmony, balanced by the pulls of the muscles involved.

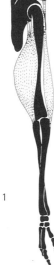

1

2

# 8 Blood

## *River of life*

Besides supporting your body and moving it, your skeletal muscles also take part in circulating your blood and lymph, in governing your body temperature and affecting your breathing. Thus, proper muscle condition will help those parts of your body over which you have no direct power. Indirect influence is also a kind of control.

*Circulation of the blood:* Your heart iself is a muscle that pumps 3,200 gallons (14,400 litres) of blood round your body every day. Your bloodstream is rightly called the river of life because of the oxygen it carries along with it.

You can live for a day or two without water, for quite a long time without food, but only a few minutes without oxygen. While most of the materials your body needs for life can be stored, oxygen has to be delivered continuously. The task of carrying out this internal breathing rests with your blood.

This is made possible because about a third of the red cells consist of haemoglobin, a protein with a remarkable capacity to combine with oxygen, which is thus carried along in the bloodstream to all parts of the body. The better your circulation the more efficiently oxygen is delivered and carbon dioxide removed.

Your heart consists of two pumps. One supplies your lungs; the other has to do six or eight times as much work pumping blood round the rest of your body. The round trip from heart to distant parts and back takes less than a minute.

### Boost for the heart

Your heart as a pump has enough pressure to take blood via your arteries to the extremities of your body, but not much more. Therefore, the return of blood to your heart via the veins depends on gravity and on your muscles and breathing acting as pumps.

*Gravity:* When you are standing up the blood being pumped along the arteries to your head and other parts above your heart goes against the force of gravity. But the force of gravity returns it along the veins. Below your heart, to your legs and feet, the arterial flow is aided by gravity, but the venous flow goes against gravity.

In upside down body positions – like the headstand or handstand, but especially the non-strenuous neck-shoulder stand and so-called plough position (see page 62) – the assistance given by the force of gravity to the arterial and venous flow is reversed. The effect of the plough position, supported by a chair to make it easier, is remarkable. It seems to calm down your body, partly because your overworked back neck muscles are lengthened and relaxed in this position.

Practising all the upside down positions increases the flow of blood from your feet, legs, pelvis and abdomen to your heart directly and mechanically through gravity. And because your neck and head are placed in a horizontal position in the neck-shoulder stand or plough position, the flow from below your heart is easy and your brain well supplied. It is like flushing your body, especially your head, with blood.

When you stand for long periods you may not give enough help to the flow of blood. If the venous return is impeded, the supply to your brain suffers. Fainting is nature's way of dealing with this by bringing your body to a horizontal position where gravity is no longer a nuisance.

*Muscles as pumps:* Muscles in your thighs, legs and feet act as pumps on your veins in order to return blood to your heart. Their contractions help to squeeze veins and move blood upwards. Your veins have at frequent intervals valves allowing blood to flow upwards towards your heart but not in the reverse direction. Consequently, any pressure exerted by your surrounding muscles causes blood to flow upwards.

Movement of your muscles in walking, sitting or standing is usually enough to squeeze blood through your veins. However, practising the recommended exercises, which improve muscle efficiency and tone, ensures that the pumping action of muscles is at its optimum.

Medical research gives numerous reasons for high blood pressure. Most of them seem beyond our responsibility. But removing obstructions by releasing tension in your muscles is within your grasp. Whatever little help cultivating these movements and positions brings, it seems worth the effort.

*Breathing as a pump:* Every breath helps to return blood to your heart. When you breathe in, the pressure in your lungs is reduced below that of the outside air. This fall in pressure also applies to your heart and the veins inside your chest cavity. They are now better able to suck in blood from veins below your diaphragm. Furthermore, the movement of your diaphragm compresses your abdominal cavity, increasing the pressure there. The veins in your abdomen are therefore compressed as they are by muscle action and the ascent of blood to your heart is further aided.

Any improvement in your breathing movement and rhythm mechanically and directly aids the venous flow of blood. And as you will see later, your breathing movement, like all other movements, depends on the action of muscles.

## Ally against bacteria

*Lymph circulation:* All cells are bathed by tissue fluid. The tissue fluid known as lymph resembles blood but contains no red corpuscles. The lymphatic tissues of your body form an essential part of your body's defence against invading agents such as protozoa, bacteria, viruses or other poisonous toxins. These agents stimulate the formation of antibodies which can destroy or neutralize the poisons.

Lymph, unlike blood, is not circulated by a central pump and its movement towards your heart depends partly on gravity, partly on compression of lymphatic vessels by muscles, and partly on suction created by the movements of your breathing. Even more than with the flow of blood, muscle actions play a vital role in the circulation of lymph.

Although you have no direct power over the circulation of blood and lymph, you have an indirect influence. You can change your posture, your shape, your movements at joints and the actions of your muscles, and thereby indirectly influence these other functions of your body.

## Keeping warm

*Maintenance of body temperature:* When your body is very cold, it goes into an interesting posture. Your limbs are flexed and your body bent forward, probably because your flexor muscles are stronger than your extensors. As muscle action always produces some heat, the purpose of the muscles contracting and shivering is to assist in maintaining normal body temperature. All the energy of your body which is converted into heat and motion is produced by your skeletal muscles. When they contract and shorten, energy is used and heat is liberated. To temper your muscles is to assist them in their role in maintaining your body temperature. The gain, no matter how small, is still significant.

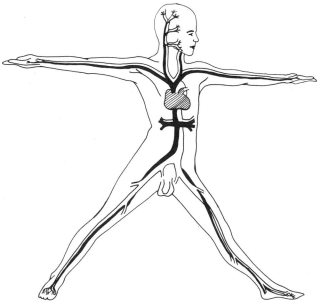

Cardiovascular system: arteries in solid, veins in outline

# 9 Breathing

## *Breath of life*

Put at its simplest, the purpose of breathing is to suck in air to provide the cells of your body with the oxygen they need and to blow out the unwanted carbon dioxide. In this complicated process two operations are involved.

The one you are aware of is breathing in and breathing out, inhaling and exhaling, your external breathing. The muscles mainly responsible for these two actions are the diaphragm, at the bottom of your chest, and the intercostal muscles between your ribs. But fully efficient breathing involves the co-ordinated activity of nearly a hundred more muscles.

Your lungs play a passive role, expanding when your diaphragm and intercostals enlarge your chest cavity and recoiling when those muscles reduce your chest cavity. The actual exchange of gases takes place in the lungs.

The delivery of oxygen to your cells is the job of another muscle – the heart – pumping oxygen-bearing blood to all parts of your body. The process of this internal breathing was outlined in the last chapter. In this chapter we are concerned with the process of external breathing and how to make it more efficient. Inadequate breathing reduces your aliveness. When your whole body takes part in your breathing your bodylife overflows.

### What you breathe with

Place your hands on your ribs, just under your breasts. Then exert a slight pressure as you exhale. Maintain the pressure and keep breathing. You will notice that you are breathing mostly with your abdomen. When you breathe abdominally, your chest muscles, temporarily unused, must rest.

Now place your hands on your abdomen, as you exhale. Hold that and breathe. Now you feel that your chest and collarbone areas are the most active.

Through doing this you have experienced those parts of your body which are directly responsible for your breathing movements. Your chest cage – ribs, breastbone and thoracic vertebrae – plus the breathing muscles – your diaphragm and intercostals – produce rhythmical, bellows-like movements, changing the capacity of your chest cavity and bringing about the inflow and expulsion of air in your lungs. The capacity of the chest cavity can be increased from side to side and from back to front by your intercostal muscles and from top to bottom by your diaphragm.

## Powerful piston

*The diaphragm*, your most important muscle in breathing, is a strong, dome-shaped sheet of muscle that lies at the bottom of your chest and roofs your abdominal cavity. When it contracts, so lengthening your chest cavity, it presses on your abdominal organs, which descend as you breathe in. When the limit of this descent is reached, your abdominal organs provide resistance to the strong central tendon of your diaphragm. The muscle part of your diaphragm then lifts up your lower ribs.

Your diaphragm, its nerves and muscles, reach into your deepest and innermost places. In its piston-like action it co-ordinates with muscles below it. Tight or overstretched abdominal muscles, front or back, connected to your lumbar vertebrae, hamper the action of your diaphragm. The front and side abdominal muscles interlace and form what is called the linea alba, which runs from the bottom of your breastbone to your pubic bones. Your abdominal muscles provide a firm but elastic wall to keep your internal organs in position and to oppose the action of gravity on them in the erect position. As they relax and contract, they take part in breathing, and their vigorous contraction is required in coughing, sneezing, vomiting, giving birth, urinating and defecating.

Your *intercostal muscles* are the muscles between your ribs and they contract when you inhale. Natural tension in these muscles prevents the interspaces of your ribs being caved in when you breathe out or ballooned out when you breathe in.

Their action increases the capacity of your ribcage, and hence the volume of your lungs. When elevated, the ends of the ribs connected to your breastbone and backbone are thrust forwards and upwards, increasing the dimension of the ribcage from front to back.

Normal breathing movements are mostly involuntary; the control centres are in the bottom part of the brain (the brain-stem) and are sensitive to impulses like the build-up of carbon dioxide in the blood. The movements are carried out automatically, that is, without conscious control, through the rhythmical discharge of nerve impulses to the muscles involved. Although the breathing centres in your brain are fundamentally automatic, and regulated by chemical factors in your blood, impulses from many parts of your body also modify the activity of these centres. Consequently, they alter the impulses that reach the muscles of breathing in order to co-ordinate rhythm, rate and depth of breathing with other activities of your body.

For example, there are interruptions of breathing out in speech and singing; deep breaths-in, then short spasmodic breaths-out, in laughter and crying; prolonged breathing out in sighing; deep breathing in, mouth open, in yawning, shallow breathing in suspense and concentration and rapid breathing in fear and excitement.

### Breathing in waves

When your body is at rest your breathing in lasts about one second and breathing out about three seconds. The physical wave associated with these movements flows from your nostrils to your genital area. If you observe carefully you can see and sense the pulsations through your own body, but they are more easily followed in the breathing of a young child.

Inhaling begins with an outward movement of the abdomen as the diaphragm contracts and abdominal muscles relax. A wave of expansion then spreads upwards to embrace the chest. Exhaling starts as a letting down in the chest and goes on as a wave of contractions to the pelvis. The whole front of the body moves in a wavelike motion, and tension in any part disturbs this natural and wavelike pattern.

*Try these tests* to see how the pattern can be disturbed.

Start by breathing while holding your chest expanded and rigid. Relax. Now breathe with your chest constricted and tight. You can still breathe, but the restriction of your breathing wave is exaggerated.

Again breathe, but this time tilt your pelvis down as far as possible with your buttocks lifted up. Freeze your pelvis in this position for a moment.

Finally breathe with your pelvis pulled up as far as possible and your abdominal muscles tight and pulled in. In both these exaggerated pelvic movements it can be seen that your breathing wave has been disturbed.

The reason is that keeping your pelvis down overstretches your abdominal muscles, while holding it tilted up over-prolongs the contraction of the muscles. The easy contraction and relaxation of abdominal muscles which is necessary for rhythmical breathing depends on your pelvis, which in turn depends on your hip joints' flexibility and support.

But your chest is also involved. A well-balanced upright position makes for a better breathing movement. And a well-balanced chest needs the free action and sound support of the thoracic vertebrae. If these are hunched together and your thoracic curve is exaggerated the movement of the chest will be restricted.

Other muscles play a part in breathing, but enough has been said to show that to breathe fully all the muscle groups in your body must be co-ordinated and in good tone. That is possible only with the support and flexibility of every joint in your body.

All the positions and movements in the book are designed to promote this flexibility. With practice you will learn to recognize the movements of your ribs, diaphragm and abdomen that make up your breathing. The better adjusted and more harmonious these movements are the deeper and easier will be your external breathing – just as we have already seen that better muscle action will improve internal breathing.

# 0 Direct relaxation

## Check list for tense muscles

Why are we so tense? When we are faced with a situation of stress our bodies prepare to act. Our primitive actions were either to fight or to flee. The rules of civilized society generally prevent this, so instead we sit and seethe. Through lack of action muscles remain tense, in a state of constant readiness, unrelaxed.

When someone tells you to relax, or when you tell yourself to do so, what does it imply? It often just means 'Stop worrying', but that soon begins to have a hollow ring when your body takes no notice of your mind's command. The more sensible approach is to go to the seat of the tension – the contracted muscles themselves.

There are tensions in your muscles of which, more likely than not, you have no direct awareness. Most people are in a state of prolonged, involuntary muscle tension from which they are unable to free themselves, even when resting or sleeping.

To show how muscle tension works against you, *try this:* Lift up the end of a heavy table. Try to think what you have done since you got up in the morning; try to carry on a conversation; try to sing. It is hard to do any of these things because of the tension demanded of your muscles. Now let the table down, and everything becomes easier.

There, in exaggerated form, is the kind of tension you have to cope with. For muscles to remain tense, energy must be used. Hence in a state of prolonged muscle contraction energy is being wasted. Chronic fatigue is the result. Wits may become dull, memory impaired and your ability to learn reduced.

On the other hand, if energy is not being wasted in keeping your neck, chest, shoulders, belly and so on rigid and tight, if it is not used up restricting movement at the joints, it can go towards improving your thinking and feeling. You become more self-contained and self-confident.

So how can you discover whether your muscles are involuntarily tense? If you suffer recurring aches frequently and your joints are stiff and inflexible, you simply are not muscularly relaxed. You may insist that you are not nervous, and you may not be. You may insist that you are aware and in control of yourself, and you may well be. You may insist that the position in which you hold your body is perfectly

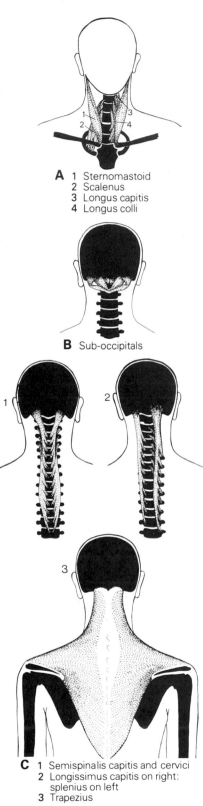

**A**
1 Sternomastoid
2 Scalenus
3 Longus capitis
4 Longus colli

**B** Sub-occipitals

**C**
1 Semispinalis capitis and cervici
2 Longissimus capitis on right:
   splenius on left
3 Trapezius

comfortable, and it probably is. But the fact remains that you are physically tense and restricted in movement at your joints. So check out your movements at each major joint of your body.

The following brief illustrated guide (although not anatomically precise) will help you to locate the major muscles working your neck, shoulders, and hips. You will then be able to take full advantage of the self-help series of movements in the second half of the book. Their purpose is to help you to learn to relax, in action and at rest, and to eliminate tensions from your body through creating movement at your joints, so as to make better use of the dynamic energy running through you and live a fuller life. Relaxation is a basic human need.

**Moving a head**

Try these head movements while pressing your fingers about your neck and its base:

1 Drop your head forward (flexion).
2 Thrust your head back as far as possible (extension).
3 Place one ear or the other close to your shoulder (lateral bending).
4 Place your chin near one or other shoulder (rotation).
5 Rotate your head clockwise and anti-clockwise (circumduction).

Now try the first four again but this time use your hand to resist the movements. The muscles involved will then speak for themselves, because resisting a movement forces the active muscles to react more powerfully. You will unmistakably feel their contraction within your own body.

These movements are mainly controlled by the numerous muscles that travel up your neck to the base of your skull. Muscles that move your head may be divided into three main groups:

1 Your front and side muscles, which consist principally of your (sternocleidomastoid) sternomastoid muscle, scalenus anterior, medius and posterior, longus colli and longus capitis. Against gravity and resistance these muscles flex your neck, also producing rotation of your head to the sides. Your sternomastoids together flex your head against gravity when your body is supine. (A)

2 Six small muscles, the sub-occipital muscles, play a part in fine skull movements. Against resistance or gravity these recti and oblique capitis muscles flex, extend, laterally flex or rotate your head according to their attachments. They act in unison with your eye muscles, causing your head to turn with your eyes. (B)

3 The last group of head-neck muscles, although concerned with movement of your head, actually extend down

into your back – with the exception of trapezius, the most superficial muscle on the back of your neck. Semispinalis capitis, longissimus capitis and splenius are attached to your head and both your cervical and thoracic vertebrae. In the erect position they act against gravity in forward flexion of your head. Your superficial trapezius can draw your head backwards and sidewards when your shoulders are fixed. (C)

All these head and neck muscles are very strong – they must be to balance and move such a weight as your skull, which is supported on a very small surface in relation to its size.

Your neck vertebrae as a unit form a universal joint, capable of movement in all directions. They can flex forward, extend backwards, move sideways to left and right, rotate or twist to left and right and circumduct. Your task is to assist these movements to their full extremity. In doing so you assist in directly lengthening and relaxing all these muscle groups.

### Action-packed shoulders

Three groups of muscles act on your shoulder girdle, joint and arm on each side of your body:

**1 The muscles connecting your upper limbs with your backbone area** are:
*Trapezius,* a pair of large flat triangular muscles which extend over the back of your neck and adjacent parts.
*Latissimus dorsi,* the very broad back muscle. (D)
*Rhomboid major* and *rhomboid minor,* two muscles connecting the last cervical vertebra and the first five thoracic vertebrae with your shoulderblade.
*Levator scapulae,* connecting the first four cervical vertebrae with your shoulderblade, which it raises. (E)

**2 The muscles connecting your upper limb and chest wall** are:
*Pectoralis major* and *pectoralis minor,* the large and small breast muscles, or pectorals. (F)
*Serratus anterior,* runs from inside your shoulderblade to your ribs.
To feel these three muscles contracting, lift your right arm to the vertical and with the other hand resist lowering your arm.

**3 The muscles connecting your shoulderblade and arm** are:
*Deltoid,* a muscle shaped like a capital delta, Δ, the Greek D.
*Subscapularis,* the muscle under your shoulderblade.
*Supraspinatus* and *infraspinatus,* the muscles above and below the spine of the shoulderblade.
*Teres minor* and *teres major,* the muscles connecting your shoulderblade to your arm bone. (G)

These three groups of muscles connecting your upper limbs

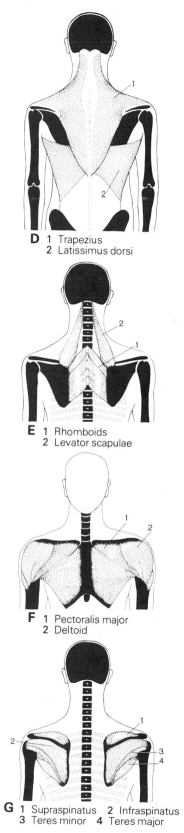

**D** 1 Trapezius
2 Latissimus dorsi

**E** 1 Rhomboids
2 Levator scapulae

**F** 1 Pectoralis major
2 Deltoid

**G** 1 Supraspinatus  2 Infraspinatus
3 Teres minor  4 Teres major

55

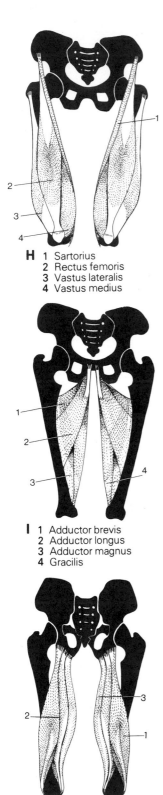

**H** 1 Sartorius
2 Rectus femoris
3 Vastus lateralis
4 Vastus medius

**I** 1 Adductor brevis
2 Adductor longus
3 Adductor magnus
4 Gracilis

**J** 1 Biceps femoris
2 Semitendinosus
3 Semimembranosus

with your chest and backbone and connecting your shoulder-blade with your arm are the muscles you should aim to contract and stretch to the full in order to balance the action of their pulls when your shoulders are at rest.

**Your heavily-worked hips**
Two principal groups of muscles act on your hip joints – the muscles of your thighs and those of your pelvis. The thigh muscles also act on your knee joints and are subdivided into three groups. The pelvis muscles also act on your sacrum and lumbar backbone and they are subdivided into inside and outside groups.

*The muscles of your thigh* are divided into front, inner and back muscles.

1  **The front thigh muscles** are:
*Sartorius*, a long, narrow muscle which crosses your thigh at a slant in front.
*Quadriceps femoris*, a four-headed muscle, comprising vastus lateralis, vastus medius and vastus intermedius, meaning immense side, middle and intermediate muscles, and rectus (straight femoris). To feel their contraction, sit with legs stretched in front of you and lift your right leg, resisting the movement with your hands. (H)

2  **The inner thigh muscles** are:
*Gracilis* which is very slender.
*Pectineus*, which starts from the ilias or comb-like part of your hip.
*Adductor longus, adductor brevis* and *adductor magnus* (long, short and large adductors). These muscles can be felt contracting by lying with your back on the floor with your legs spread apart against a wall, then bringing your feet together and resisting the movement with your hands. (I)

3  **The back thigh muscles (the hamstring group)** are:
*Biceps femoris*, the two-headed thigh muscle.
*Semitendinosus* and *semimembranosus*, the half-tendon muscle and half-membrane muscle. These muscles can be felt contracting by lying on your back, lifting your right leg and then resisting the movement downwards. Hold your hands cupped behind your upper back thighs. (Why it is so important to relax your hamstring muscles? The answer is simply that by assisting your body to bend fully at your hip joints you have relaxed the largest, strongest and probably the hardest-worked muscle group in your body.) (J)

*The muscles of the pelvis* are:
1  **The articular muscles,** which connect the hip joint and thigh to the inside of the pelvis or hips: they are:
*Obturator internus* and *externus;*

*Gemilli;*
*Piriformis;*
*Quadratus femoris.*

2 **The gluteal muscles,** which are on the outside of the hips and connect the hip joints to the pelvis and lower back. They are:
*Gluteus maximus, gluteus medius* and *gluteus minimus,* usually known as the buttock muscles. (K1 & K2)
*Tensor fasciae latae,* which stretches the side fascia. To feel this muscle contracting, sit with your legs stretched in front of you and take your right leg to the right, resisting the movement with your right hand.

3 **The iliac muscles,** which connect to the hip joint, pelvis and lower back. They are:
*Psoas major* and *psoas minor, muscles of the loin; iliacus,* the muscle of the top hip bone or ilium. (L1 & L2)

These six groups of muscles on each side of your body act on your hip joints. The three thigh groups on each side also act on your knee joints, while the three pelvic groups on each side act on your sacrum and lumbar joints. Your aim is to ensure that the muscles are capable of *fully* contracting and *fully* relaxing, so ensuring that at rest your hips balance in alignment on your thigh bones and your backbone balances on your pelvis. Movements and positions will be given to help you do just this.

### Best foot forward and backward
Your ankle is a true hinge joint which enables you to bend your foot either forwards (plantar-flexion) or backwards (dorsi-flexion) and very little else.

*Try this:* Sit down with your legs straight in front of you. Now resist with your hand the movement of bringing your foot backwards to your leg. Note which muscles are felt contracting. Then resist plantar-flexing your foot, that is, pointing your toes. Again, note which muscles contract. In those two resisted movements you have felt all the muscle groups that operate your ankle.

The muscle lengthened and relaxed in pointing the foot is called tibialis anterior (see page 58). It is situated in front of your shin bone. When your foot is on the ground, the front shin bone muscle helps to keep the balance of your body by pulling your leg forwards upon your foot at your ankle joint and also assists in pulling your leg inwards. When your foot is free, it actively dorsi-flexes your foot. It is more frequently affected in polio than any other muscle, and its deterioration results in a drop-foot gait.

The main muscle lengthened and relaxed in dorsi-flexing your foot is the back shin bone muscle, tibialis posterior. When your foot is on the ground this muscle pulls your leg

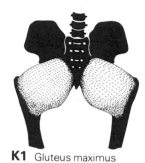

**K1** Gluteus maximus

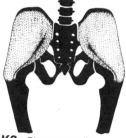

**K2** Gluteus medius

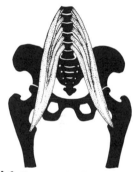

**L1** Psoas major & minor

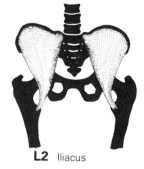

**L2** Iliacus

backwards in adjusting the balance of your body and also pulls it inwards. Its most important function is that of being the strongest support of the long arch of your foot. When your foot is free it points your foot at your ankle joint.

Two other muscles, peroneus longus and brevis, take part in balancing your body, pulling your leg outwards when your foot is on the ground. With your foot free they assist in pointing it.

In the erect position your calf muscles (soleus and gastrocnemius) are continually engaged in keeping your balance because the centre of gravity passes in front of your ankle joint. Connected to your heel by the six-inch-long achilles tendon, they are the most powerful plantar-flexors, keeping you on your toes and physically alert, and are among the main driving forces in locomotion, from walking to running, dancing and jumping.

Very frequently these muscles cannot relax sufficiently to permit full dorsi-flexion at the ankle joint. Most people who have worn high-heeled shoes for any length of time are restricted in dorsi-flexion because the calf muscles have shortened and stiffened with continual contraction.

To relax, lengthen and tone your leg and ankle muscles, you need only assist plantar-flexion and dorsi-flexion of the foot to their extreme maximum. Through cultivation and practice of these two movements you will gain or regain the ability fully to contract and lengthen all the muscles operating your ankle joints.

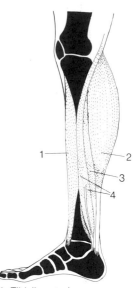

1 Tibialis anterior
2 Gastrocnemius
3 Soleus
4 Peroneus brevis & longus

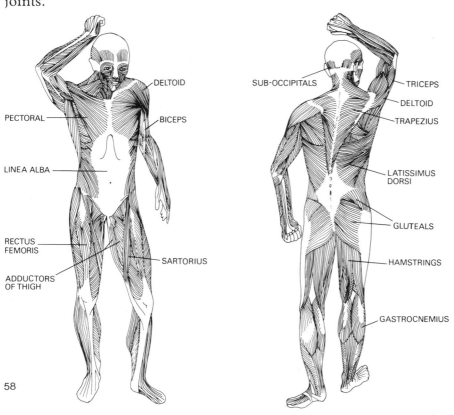

SUB-OCCIPITALS
TRICEPS
DELTOID
TRAPEZIUS
LATISSIMUS DORSI
GLUTEALS
HAMSTRINGS
GASTROCNEMIUS

DELTOID
PECTORAL
BICEPS
LINEA ALBA
RECTUS FEMORIS
SARTORIUS
ADDUCTORS OF THIGH

58

# PART 2  11 The ground rules: questions and answers

Before you start the movements here are answers to some of the questions that are likely to come into your mind.

### Are the movements safe?
First of all, explain to your doctor the exercises you are planning to do, so that he can tell you whether you have any ailment that could be worsened by exercise.

The movements themselves are neither spectacular nor unusual. Many of them are prescribed by specialists in physical medicine and therapies. Others come from very ancient ways of conditioning the body. Each person's body is unique, so each person will vary in his or her ability to carry out the movements. But everyone must carry out the programme gradually. There is no instant way to relax your body.

There are movements suitable for children, backache sufferers, the elderly and for pregnant women. Women are advised not to practise any inverted positions during their menstrual period.

### What are the movements meant to do to me?
By improving the strength and flexibility of your muscles and joints you will create a strong, flexible and relaxed body. You are not trying to develop more powerful muscle groups, but rather to relax and harmonize them. But it is harder to learn to relax than it is to develop strength. If you are strong some of these positions and movements may seem sissy to you, but you may be tense as well as strong, and these therapeutic movements will make you relax. If you are weak they will strengthen you.

Some women are so supple that they find it easy to flop into many of the positions. But they often find proper head or hand balance difficult, and if so they should concentrate on balancing positions.

Of the greatest importance is the way in which the movements will increase your awareness of your body – your sense of proprioception. Learning in this way about your body and discovering new sensations in your movements is actually great fun. As your body becomes more alive you enjoy it more.

### What equipment do I need?
For these movements your body is its own gymnasium

equipment. You have your own weight, pressure and momentum, plus the force of gravity. In these positions gravity is made to work on your side. Only when your own weight is not enough do you call on outside assistance, such as can be given by a cushion, a chair, a wall and occasionally another person.

For a work-out the less you wear the better, but whatever you choose it should be comfortable.

### When should I do the movements?
There are two answers to that.

Some of the movements require that you set aside half an hour each day for them. Make this a time when you will *never* be disturbed. You owe this to yourself. We give so much time and attention to other things in life. Your body muscles and joints need them as well, sometimes desperately.

There are many other movements which can be done at almost any time of the day, at work, on a bus, in a lift, and so on. For instance, when you are driving and the car is stopped at a red light bend your head sideways to rest it on each shoulder alternately. At the end of the day you will have done this movement many times without having had to put aside a special time for it.

If you think you are too irritated to face a work-out remember that the time when you feel harried and put down is when you need the movements most, because you are doing them to release tension. Excessive tension, or prolonged contraction that your muscles have built up during a hectic day, can be released through these movements and positions.

For the half-hour you are doing them make nothing more important than the job in hand. And as you live one day at a time so work one session at a time.

If you like, you can bathe before a work-out – or after, or before and after, or indeed neither.

### How much time should I spend on each movement?
Very little at the start, building up very, very gradually until the movement becomes easy. Suggested times are given in the detailed instructions, where you will find constant warnings that you should stay in a position only as long as you find it comfortable. To go on longer is to miss the point. These are not lessons in sheer effort, but in how to turn strenuous movements into easy ones. Use caution and take notice of any painful alarm signals.

### Will the exercises hurt me, then?
As was explained in the chapter on making friends with pain (Chapter 3), in the process of restoring flexibility to your body pain which has been suppressed may surface again. This is the pain that comes from releasing the rigidity of muscles. It is beneficial pain.

It is important to recognize during the movements which pains are signals of harmful stress and strain and which are beneficial pains. If you stretch a muscle that is already overstretched you experience a harmful pain that is telling you to stop. If you move a joint further off-centre than it is already, the resulting pain is a demand that you should do something about it. However, if you stretch a short, chronically contracted muscle the resulting pain is like that experienced when blood flows back into a frozen finger, making it feel more alive afterwards. It is beneficial pain.

You may be avoiding pain at present by not attempting movements that once you could do and would dearly love to be able to do again. So getting rid of the limitations on your movements instead of weakly accepting them is likely to be rather painful at first. Gradually you learn to do the movements correctly, your body adjusts and the pain goes.

**How long will it take me to master all the positions?**
That is the wrong question. Doing the movements in the way described is more important for the improvement of your posture than merely achieving the final position. The exercises are devised to benefit your body as a whole through acting on its various parts. If you wanted merely to achieve the final positions you could probably produce the desired movements by distorting your body, but there is no sense or virtue in that.

If in every movement you remain aware of your body as a whole, you will make that movement at its proper source and there will be no distortion, even if one result is that you have not made the full movement or reached the final position.

All the movements must be performed slowly and smoothly. Do not make jerky movements. Do not strain. Do not force. Be sure to rest for a while between each exercise. Speed and rhythm come much later when your body is strong and supple.

Accept the fact that trying to get back to par from below par is by no means easy, but it is foolish going bull-headed at the exercises solely to achieve the final positions.

One last word of advice – about breathing. Breathe normally. If you find yourself holding your breath, consciously try to resume normal breathing. Take note of your breathing in every movement, but do not interfere or try to control it. Regular practice of this will result quite naturally in a calming and deepening of the breath.

With the workings of the body explained, the purpose of the movements set out and the ground rules established, you are now well prepared to start work on the self-help programme that makes up the rest of the book.

# 12 Flexibility

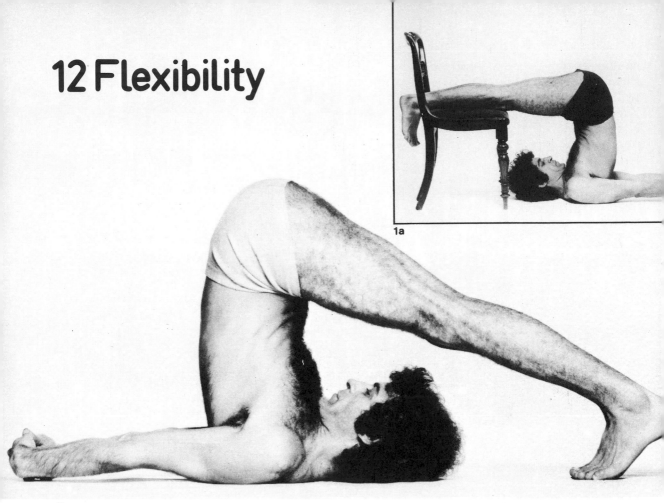

1a

1b

## *Neck and shoulder movements*

Both are intimately involved in any shoulder action, as you will appreciate if you hold your neck between your hands and then shrug your shoulders several times. For your neck muscles to be relaxed, your shoulder muscles must be relaxed.

**Movement 1: To flex your neck fully**
Take a stool with a cushion on it. Lie down with your head a foot or so away. Bend your knees and with your hands as support lift your trunk off the ground. Then slowly straighten your legs until they rest on the stool (**1a**). Hold this position for about half a minute. With practice you should gradually be able to remain in it with ease for 5 minutes. In this position you use the weight and leverage of your trunk and legs to lengthen the overworked muscles at the back of your neck. When this position has become easy try extending your arms backwards with hands interlocked. This lengthens your shoulder and breast muscles.

The final stage (**1b**) is to do it without the stool.

## Movement 2: To extend your neck fully

Place a mat or a thick folded blanket on a solid table against a wall. Lie on your back, buttocks against the wall. Flex your knees with your feet on the wall. Let your head hang over the edge of the table with your arms by your sides as in the photograph. Stay like this for half a minute and build up to 5 minutes.

The point is to ensure that your back stays flat on the table. Keep your lower jaw closed against your upper jaw. Do not open your mouth, or you will not get the proper throat stretch. Your throat and front neck muscles are lengthened with assistance from gravity, and without resistance, strain or stress on your lower back.

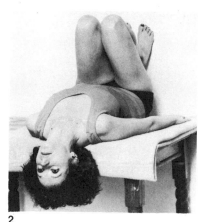

2

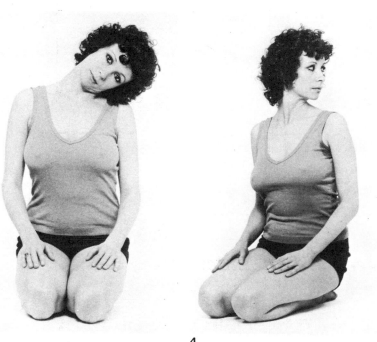

3                                    4

## Movement 3: To bend your neck sideways

Sitting or standing, keep your chin slightly in and at the centre line of your body. Now gently place your ear as near as possible to your right shoulder. Lengthen your neck as your head goes down. This movement lengthens the trapezius muscle of the opposite side. Now do the same on the left. It can be done many times a day.

## Movement 4: To rotate your head

Centre your head with chin very slightly in and rotate your head first to the left and then to the right, as if you were trying to look behind you. Hold on each side for a few seconds, gently rotating as much as possible. This too can be done many times every day.

## Movement 5: To extend your arms overhead

Lie on your back with your legs on a wall, forming an L with your trunk and legs. Now bend your knees as much as possible, with your feet against the wall. With your fingers interlocked, take your arms overhead, keeping your elbows straight and firm (**5a**). Lie in this position for a minute and build up to 5 or 10 minutes.

You can also use the momentum of your arms by raising them and then swinging them on to the floor in rhythm with your breathing. If your breast muscles are tight, your arms will not make complete contact with the floor. With practice, they should be able to lie flat on the floor along their entire length. When they do so effortlessly, your breast muscles are sufficiently long and relaxed.

Try the same position on a table against a wall. This allows your arms to go beyond 180 degrees. Make sure your elbows are straight. Your head should rest on the edge of the table (**5b**). Stay in this position for a minute and build up to 5 or 10 minutes.

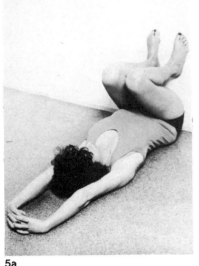

5a

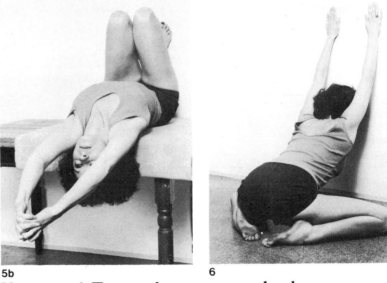

5b    6

## Movement 6: To extend your arms overhead

This position relaxes the same muscles as the last movement. Sit on your feet with knees apart, or on the floor with knees apart (or on the edge of a chair), a few feet away from a wall. Your elbows should be straight and your hands about shoulder width apart.

Here you use the weight of your body against the wall to lengthen your front shoulder muscle groups. Don't force, rather let go and relax. Start at 1 minute and build up to 5. You can also do this in rhythm with your breathing. Sit up straight on inhalation and extend on to the wall on exhalation.

**Movement 7: To rotate your arms outwards fully**
Sitting comfortably on the floor, or standing, extend your arms
out to your sides, with palms facing downwards. Now bring
your palms upwards and backwards so that both arms rotate as
far as they can. Hold for 5 seconds and relax. Repeat this as
many times in a day as you wish. To check your progress, bend
your elbow the first time you do this, using your hand as a
pointer. Then recheck in a month or so.

**Movement 8: To rotate your arms outwards**
Sitting or standing, bend your elbows at right angles. Keep
your elbows close to your body and gently swing your hands
outwards. Let the momentum build up until the swing out
actually stretches your breast and shoulder muscles. This
movement may be done by clapping your hands in front of your
body, then swinging outwards as far as possible, keeping your
elbows close to your body. It may be done as many times as you
wish.

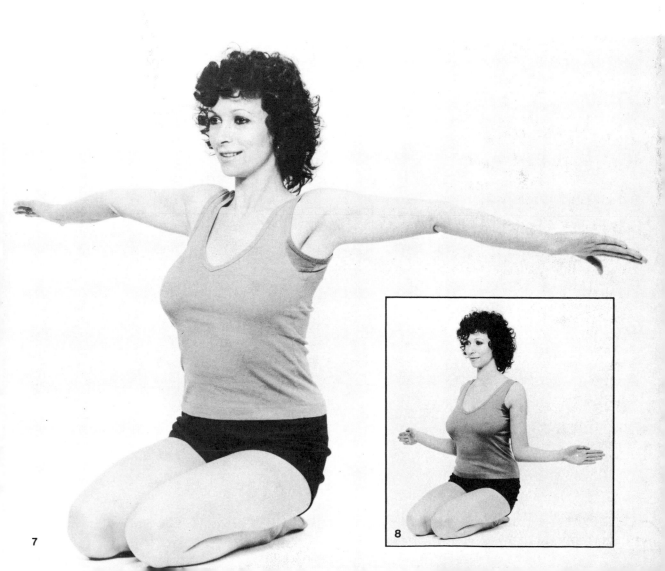

**Movement 9: To extend your arms backwards fully**
Sitting on your feet bend forward with arms going backwards
as far as possible and hands interlocked. Ask someone to assist
the movement – just a gentle pull. (If you pull your arms back
towards your buttocks against resistance, you will feel which
muscles contract. These are the groups of muscles which are
relaxed and lengthened in this movement.)

**Movement 10: Interlocking your hands on your back**
Sitting, take one hand overhead, bending your arm backwards
to meet the other arm going down and backwards. Repeat with
hands reversed.

**Movement 11: Palm in palm on your back**
Take both hands behind your back so that your palms face
each other. Take your elbows backwards and keep your trunk
straight. Do not arch your back.

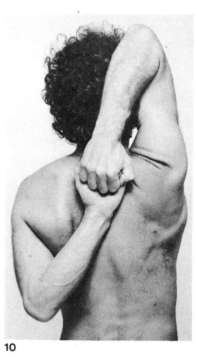

10

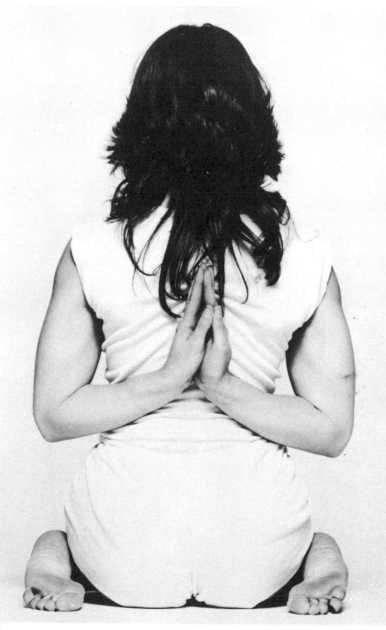

11

# Hip joint, knee and ankle movements

All these exercises, standing, sitting and lying down, are designed to make your hip joints, knees and ankles more flexible – only six joints, but the muscles of your buttocks, thighs and legs are the largest and strongest in your body. To get them to recover their ability to lengthen and shorten to the full is no simple challenge. Do not rush. The longer you take the better. You are dealing with your own body.

**Check list for standing exercises**
Standing erect is the starting point for all the standing positions and most of your everyday movements. When you stand ready to begin each movement, make this quick check:

Your head should be level, not tilted backwards, forwards or sideways.

Your shoulders should lie lightly, not braced, pulled forward or raised.

Your breathing should be easy, with a gentle abdominal movement along with the movement of your chest.

Your pelvis should be level, neither tucked in nor stuck out.

Your legs should be straight, without rigidly bracing your knees.

Your weight should fall evenly over your feet, that is, on two heels and two soles.

If all these are correct, your backbone will be upright without being braced or stiff – just as it should be.

**Movement 12: Standing – forward bending of pelvis and trunk**
Standing with your feet about a foot apart, bend forward with your hands joined on your buttocks. Lever your pelvis and trunk from as far back as your hip bones (**12a**).

Keep your body, from your buttock bones to your head, as straight and relaxed as possible. Do not bend your neck. For the best leverage, lift your shoulderblades lightly towards your hands. Use the weight of your trunk as a lever to lengthen the back muscles of both your legs. The final position is with your lower abdomen and chest on your thighs, but do not try to get there at any cost; achieve it gradually. Begin with half a minute at a time, and build up to 5 or 10 minutes.

You can effectively use the weight of your body to lengthen the back of one limb at a time by slightly flexing the other limb (**12b**).

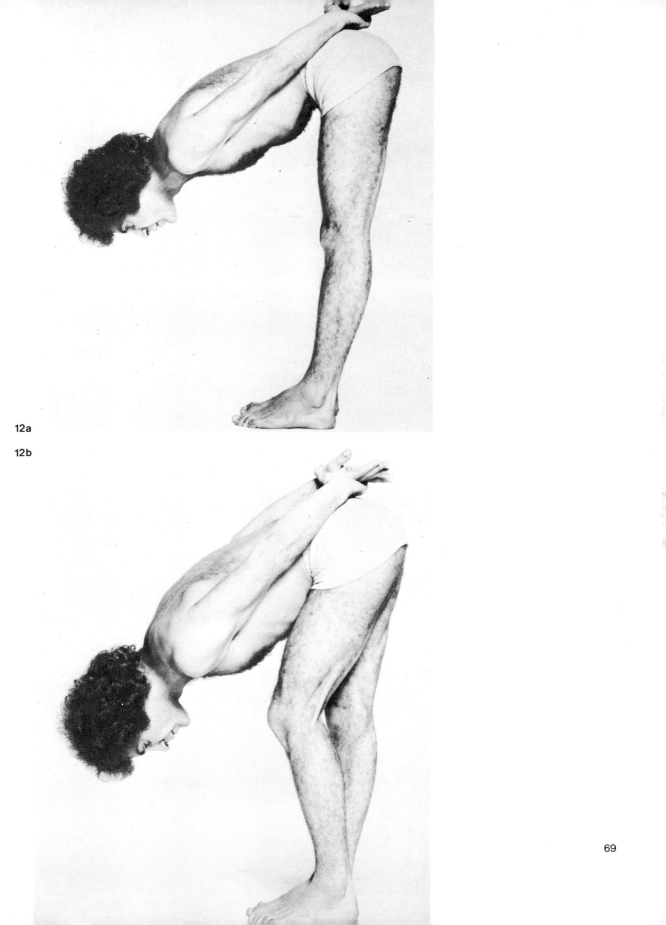

12a

12b

69

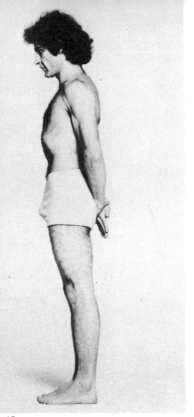

Another approach is to bend forward in rhythm, breathing out as you go down, breathing in as you come up. Here you use the momentum of your body to stretch your back thighs (**12c-f**).

There should be very little movement of your head, neck, trunk and shoulders as you lever from your buttocks. When you can hang well forward with ease, then use your hands to complete the movement (**12g**). The most common fault is overbending (**12h**) the trunk because of tight hamstrings and lack of movement in the pelvis.

**Final position (12i)**
Feet together, knees fully extended, entire front of trunk on thighs. Lift buttocks as high as possible.

12c

12d

12e

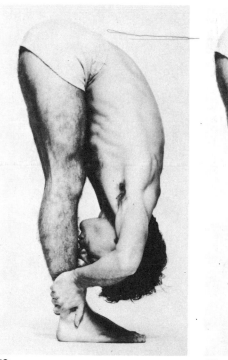

12g

12h

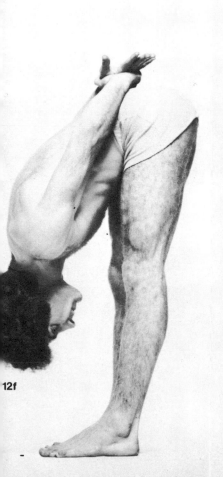

12f

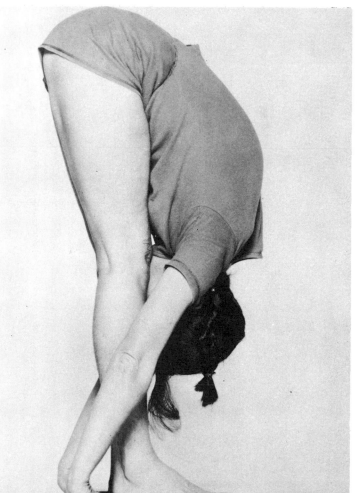

12i

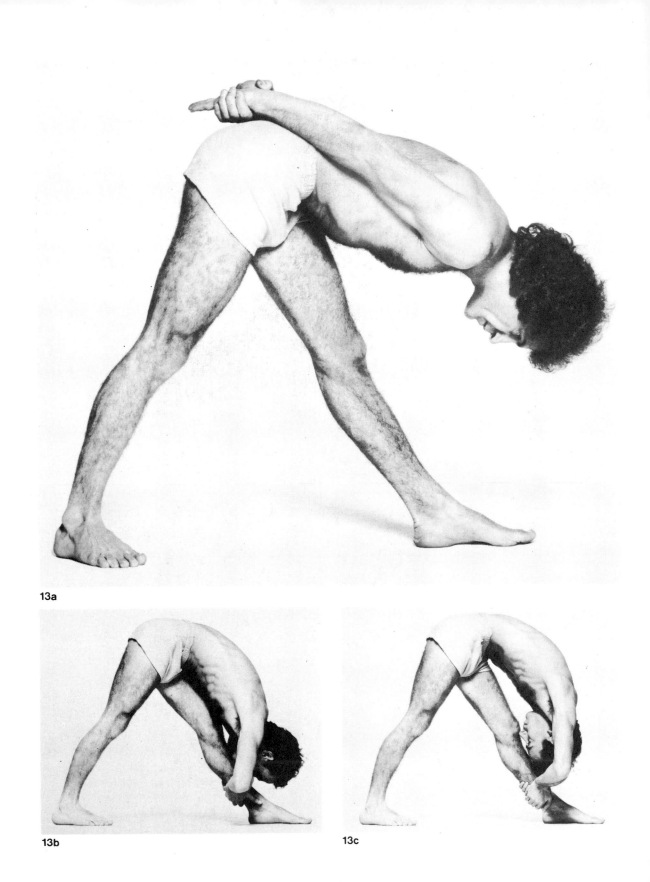

13a

13b

13c

## Movement 13: Bending pelvis and trunk forward, one leg forward, one backward

From a starting position, with feet together, move your left foot 18 inches forward and your right foot 18 inches backward, back toes out at 45 degrees. With your hands joined on your buttocks, slowly lever your pelvis and trunk to bend forward from your buttock bones, as far as is comfortable (**13a**). Your head, trunk and pelvis should be straight but relaxed. Try to let your pelvis and trunk hang forward. Repeat on the other side. Begin with half a minute on each side and build up to 3 minutes.

The principal stretch is behind your front knee. To add an extra stretch to your hamstrings, lift the front of your front foot off the floor with your weight on your heel. As with the previous movement, the most common fault is overbending your trunk (**13c**). **13b** shows the correct position.

### Final position (13d)
Allow trunk to go forward from pelvis with no strain on back. Lift buttock bones as high as possible. Abdomen and chest should touch the front thigh. Knees should be straight, and neck and head relaxed.

### Variations (13e,f)
**13e** Fingers interlocked and arms extended backwards.
**13f** Hands behind back, palm to palm.

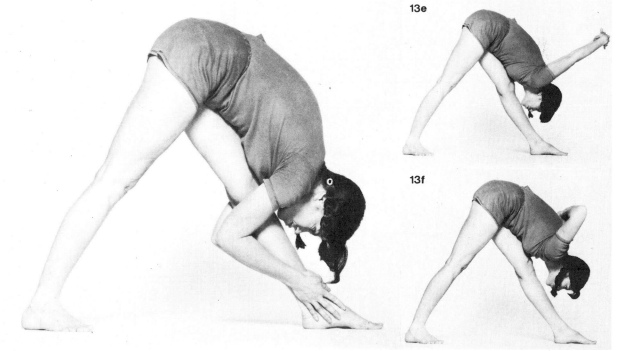

13e

13f

13d

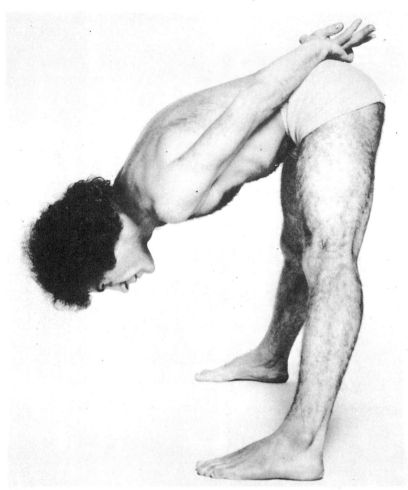

**14a**

## Movement 14: Bending pelvis and trunk forward with feet apart

Spread your feet 5 feet apart, your heels out and your toes slightly in. With your hands joined on your buttocks, lever your pelvis and trunk forward, bending from your buttock bones (**14a**). Just hang comfortably, without applying any effort. Keep your pelvis, trunk and head in a straight line.

This lengthens and relaxes your back and inner thigh muscles.

Build up the time from half a minute to 3 or 5 minutes. When your movement forward is easier, grip your ankles and lever further forward (**14b**). Again, the most common fault is overbending the trunk and not lifting up the buttock bones (**14d**). **14c** shows the correct position.

### Final position (14e)

Bend forward from pelvis, with buttocks as high as possible. Trunk and head should be as straight and relaxed as possible.

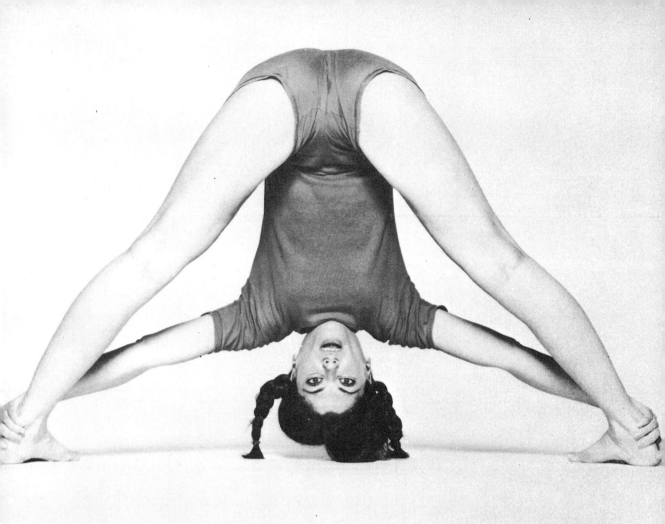

**14b**

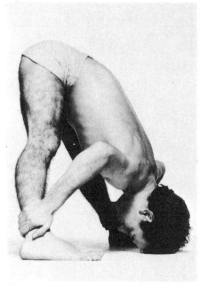

**14c**

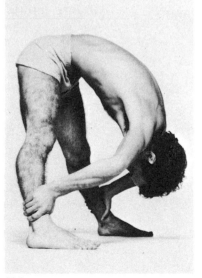

**14d**

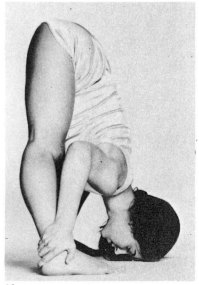

**14e**

When your hamstrings have lengthened and relaxed sufficiently, you may try the next position, but do not force it.

## Movement 15: Forward bend of pelvis and trunk with leg extended backwards

**15a** As pelvis and trunk come forward, back leg is lifted as high as possible. Hands on floor help to keep balance. Repeat on other side.

**15b** Use one hand to pull trunk to leg and the other to help to keep balance. Repeat on other side.

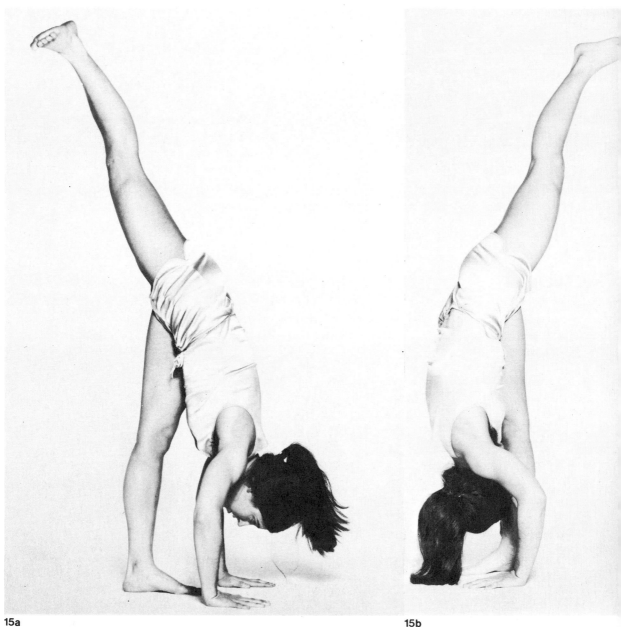

15a                                                    15b

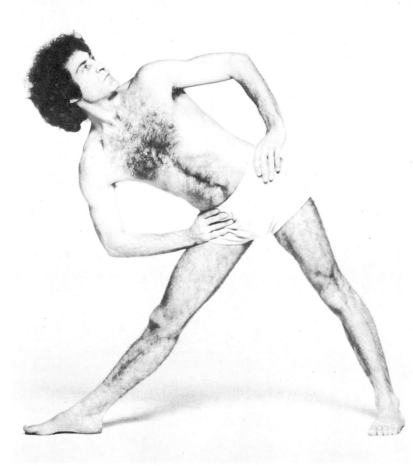

16b

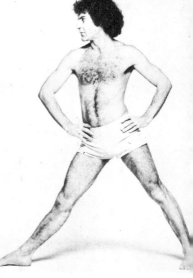

16a

## Movement 16: Sideways bending of pelvis and trunk

With your hands on your hips, spread your legs apart about the length of one of your legs, so that the distance between your feet and your two legs make up an equilateral triangle. Turn the right foot 90 degrees to the right, pointing straight, and the left slightly inwards to the right. Align your feet so that an imaginary line runs from your front foot through the heel to the middle of your back foot (**16a**). Now take your hips on to the back leg as far as possible, inclining your trunk slightly to the right; then lever your hips and trunk to your right side as much as you can without strain (**16b**). Just lower them enough to be still comfortable. The source of the bending is mainly at your hip joints, so avoid caving in your lower chest by bending your trunk. Make sure your trunk is directly above your front leg, not in front or behind it. Do not tilt your pelvis down; keep it straight to ensure that your lower back is curved as little as possible. Check that your front knee turns outwards so that the arch of your foot is lifted and your foot is not flat. Repeat the same on the other side.

In this exercise you lever the weight of your pelvis and trunk in order to lengthen and relax your back thigh muscles. You may practise it as many times a day as you can.

To get extra length, lift the ball of your front foot off the ground, putting your weight on the heel.

The principal mistake most people make is to bend the trunk and so cramp the lower ribs (**16d**), instead of bending from the pelvis at the hip joints (**16c**).

After you have cultivated this side movement with your hands on your hips, try making the same movement but with your arms extended and rotated, palms upwards and backwards. Eventually, you will touch the floor.

### Final position (16e)
Weight on outside of feet. Knees straight. Front knee turning slightly out to lift inner ankle and arch. Bend at hip joints. Lower ribs should not be cramped. Turn head to look at top hand. Arms rotating outwards. Push pelvis towards back leg as much as possible. Repeat on other side.

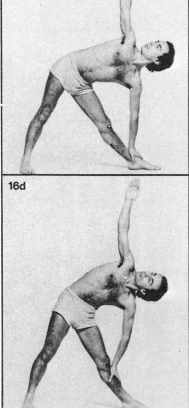

16c

16d

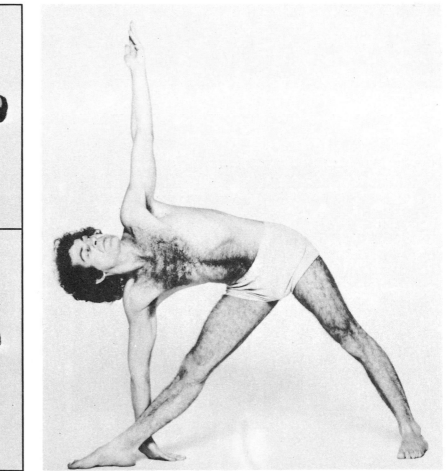

16e

## Movement 17: Sideways bending of pelvis and trunk on one leg

Supporting your back against a wall, in the final position of the previous movement, place your palm about a foot away from your front foot by bending your front knee and bringing your back foot nearer to your front one (**17a**). Raise your back leg and straighten out your supporting leg. Your trunk and back leg should be parallel to the floor. Rotate your back leg and take back your top hip so that it almost touches the wall. Don't point your toes, rather point your foot towards your knee. The knee of your supporting leg should turn outwards to the wall so as to lift your inner ankle and arch (**17b**). Repeat on the other side. When this is easy, try it without the wall.

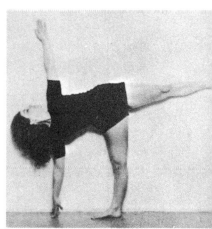

17b

## Final position (17c)

Trunk and leg parallel to floor. Back foot and leg rotating upwards. Supporting leg straight, with knee turned slightly outwards. Trunk relaxed but firm. Neck in line with trunk. Head looking at hand.

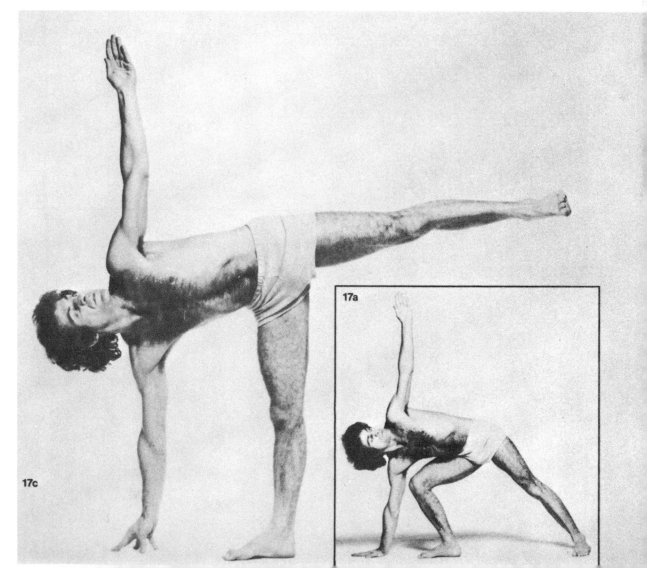

17c

17a

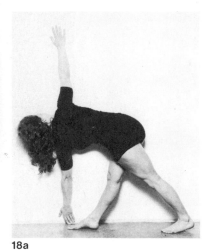

18a

## Movement 18: Rotating and bending pelvis and trunk

With your back about 4 inches away from a wall spread your feet about 3 feet apart. Turn your right foot 90 degrees to the right and your left foot 60 degrees to the right. Rotate your hips, trunk and back leg to face the wall squarely. Raise your arms sideways in line with your shoulders. Place your arms and chest squarely against the wall, then slowly lower your pelvis and trunk as far as comfortable. The stretch is felt principally behind your front leg (**18a**). Repeat on the other side.

When this movement comes easily and your palms rest on the floor, try it without the wall. The main mistake most people make in this movement is not turning the back leg in enough and rotating it (**18c**). This prevents the hips and trunk from rotating fully. (**18b**) is a better movement.

## Final position (18d)

Back foot and knee turned well inwards. Thighs as close together as possible. Lift top hip. Drop bottom hip. Chest relaxed. Trunk rotated. Head looking at top hand. Arms extended and rotated.

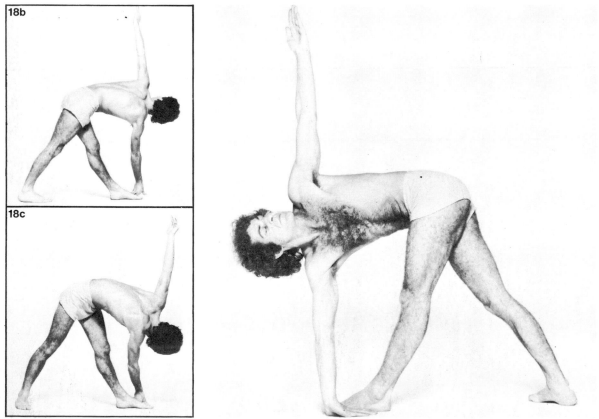

18b

18c

18d

## Movement 19: Martial Stance One

With your hands on your hips spread your feet about 5 feet apart. Turn the right foot sideways 90 degrees to the right, and the left foot slightly to the right. Keep your knees straight and the weight on the outside of your feet (**19a**). Now bend your right knee (**19b**) till your thigh is parallel to the floor and your lower leg vertical, with the knee directly above the ankle. Shift your foot forward or backward to find this position. This bending of your knee should be done without disturbing your pelvis and trunk and without your trunk inclining forward. Make sure your back knee is fully extended and your back foot firmly on the ground. Keep your front knee and thigh, hips and back leg in a straight line. Repeat on the other side.

When this becomes easy, try it with your arms extended, palms facing upwards and rotating backwards.

### Final position (19c)

Front thigh parallel to floor. Front lower leg vertical to floor. Weight on outside of feet. Keep back knee straight. Pelvis and trunk straight up as far as possible. Avoid exaggerating lower back curve. Arms extended and rotating upwards. Repeat on other side.

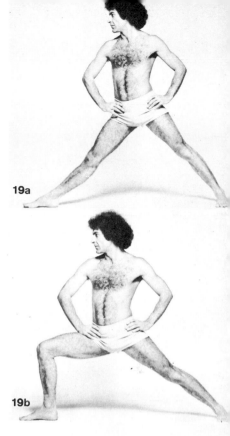

19a

19b

19c

## Movement 20: Variation of Martial Stance One

From the last position, bend your trunk sideways and place your palm on the floor beside your foot. The side of your trunk should be in contact with your thigh. Check that your back knee is extended and your back foot firmly on the floor (**20a**). Extend your other arm over your ear (**20b**) and turn your head to look at your shoulder. Your front knee and thigh, pelvis and back leg should be in a straight line. Finally, rotate your back knee, pelvis and trunk slightly outwards. Repeat on the other side.

The most common fault is overbending the trunk (**20c**) and not resting it on the front thigh.

### Final position (20d)

Palm on floor outside front foot. Avoid letting pelvis face floor. Back knee extended fully. Trunk contacting front thigh. Extend other arm over ear. Repeat on other side.

20a

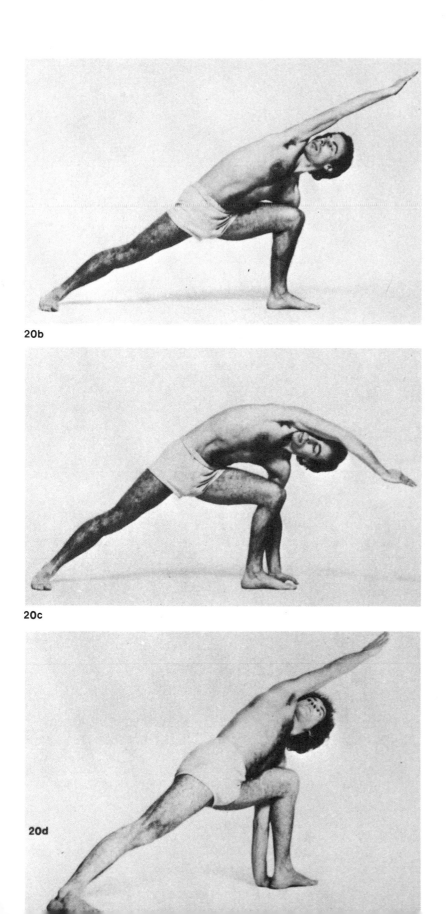

20b

20c

20d

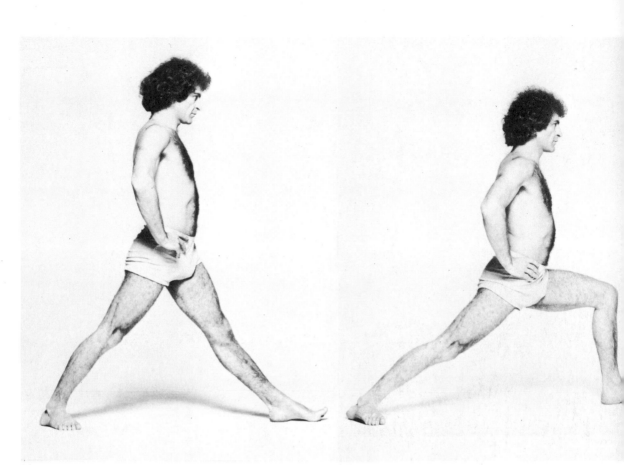

21a
21b

### Movement 21: Martial Stance Two

Stand with your feet together, facing squarely to the left, hands on your hips. Take your left foot forwards about 2½ feet and your right foot backwards the same distance. The back foot should be turned inwards about 45 degrees. Try to keep your pelvis and trunk facing the front as squarely as possible, keeping your back knee extended (**21a**). Now bend your front knee (**21b**) till your thigh is parallel to the floor and your lower leg vertical. Make sure your pelvis does not tilt downwards and exaggerate your lower back curve. Repeat on the other side.

The most common faults are not placing the front lower leg vertical to the floor and not bringing the pelvis as square to the front as possible. When this position is easy, try it with your arms extended overhead, elbows fully extended.

### Final position (21c,d)

Weight on outside of feet. Back foot and knee turned inwards. Back knee straight. Front thigh parallel to floor, and lower leg vertical to it. Pelvis square to the front. The least lower back curve possible. Arms extended overhead. Neck relaxed and head facing straight ahead. Repeat on other side.

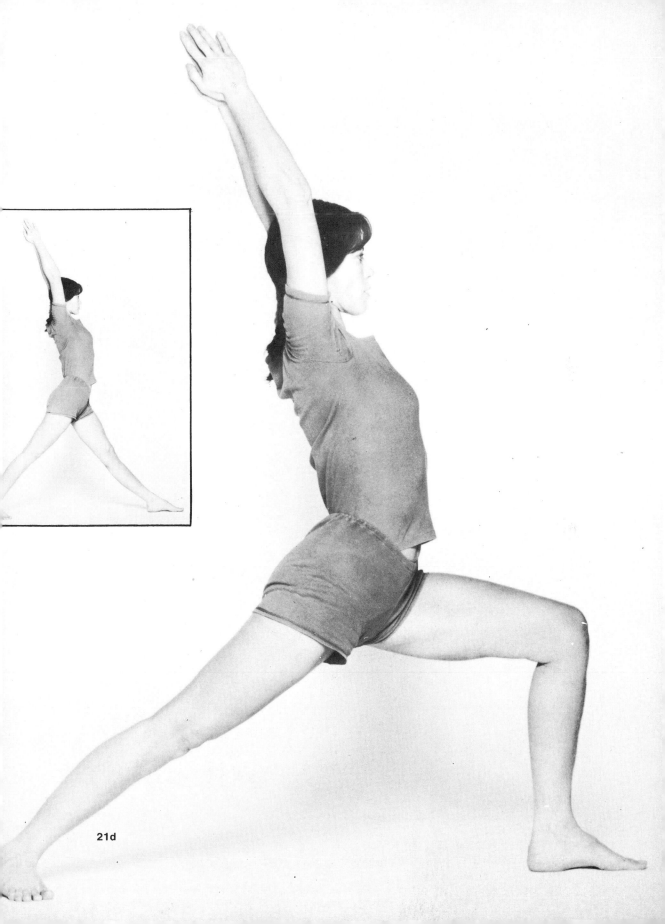

21d

## Movement 22: Continuation of Martial Stance Two

Begin this position with the help of a stool. Keep your trunk and back leg parallel to the floor. Your trunk should be as straight as possible and your back leg facing the floor to keep your pelvis level (**22a**).

When this becomes easy try the following:

From Martial Stance Two bend your trunk forward to rest on your front thigh (**22b**). Rest a few seconds, then straighten up your supporting leg as you lift your trunk and back leg (**22c**).

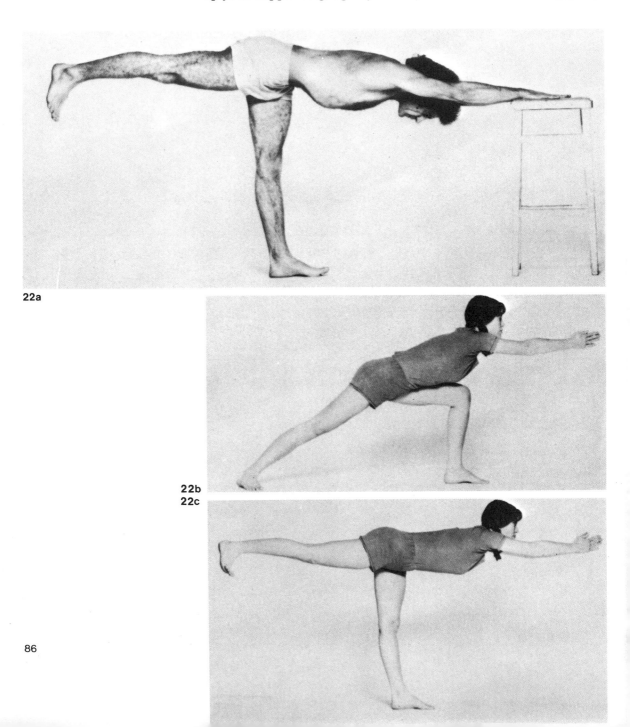

22a

22b
22c

## Movement 23: Squatting
Find something that can support the full weight of your body. Hold on to it with feet apart and gradually go into a squatting position. Build up your time gradually till you can do this with ease. Then bring your feet closer together until you can do it with feet together (**23a**).

After this stage, try it without support; again begin with feet apart and work up to feet together.

**23a**

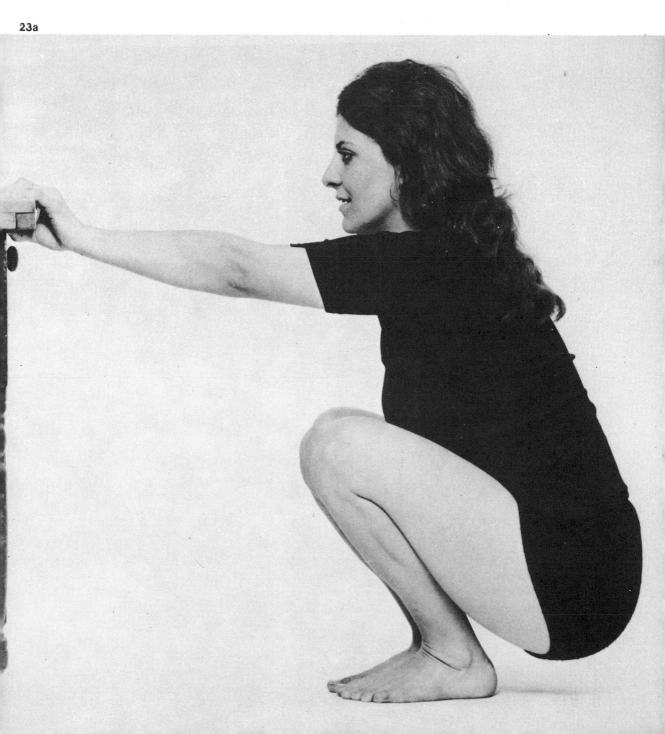

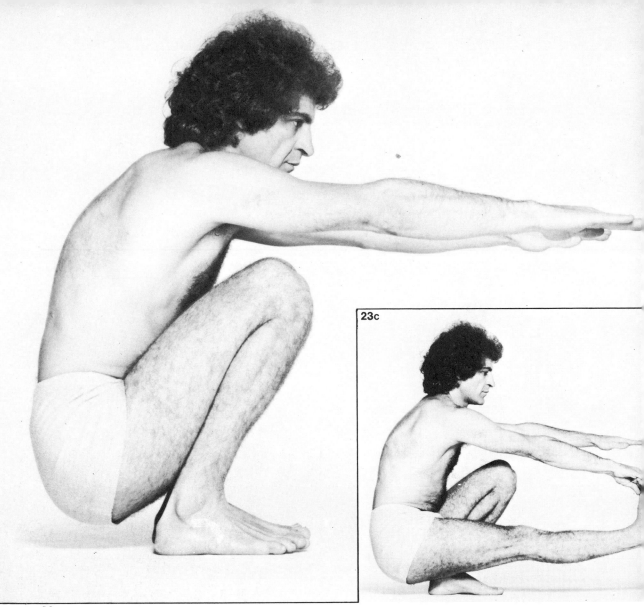

23c

23b

**Final position** (23b)
Feet together. Heels on floor. Weight on outside of feet. Arms parallel to ground.

When squatting has become easy, try these variations:

**Variation One** (23c)
Extend leg and grip big toe. Repeat on other side.

**Variation Two** (23d,e,f)
Supporting heel on ground. Extended knee facing upwards, foot pointing to knee. Cross over to other side.

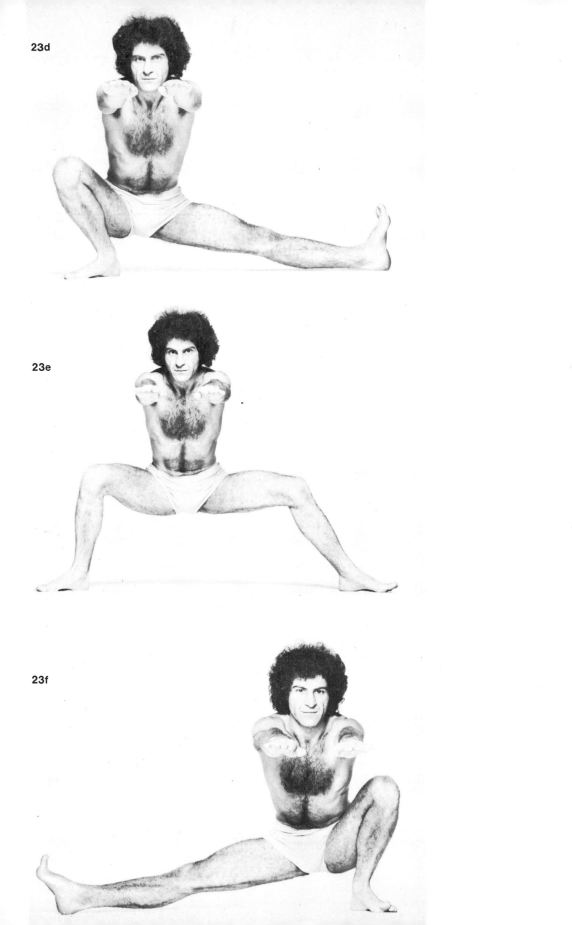

23d

23e

23f

## Movement 24: The dog position

Kneel down on the floor. Place your palms about 4 feet in front of you on the floor, the width of your shoulders apart. Now take your heels on to the floor and at the same time straighten your knees. Lift your buttocks and take your head and trunk downwards towards the floor (**24a**).

This position especially lengthens and relaxes your heel and calf muscles. You use the weight of your body to stretch them.

### Final position (24a)

Elbows and shoulders extended as much as possible. Chest moves towards the floor. Trunk extended. Stretch heels on to floor.

### Variation One (24b)

Lift leg and place on opposite side. Entire weight on extended foot. Repeat on other side.

### Variation Two (24c)

Lift extended leg as high as possible. Knee facing floor. Repeat on other side.

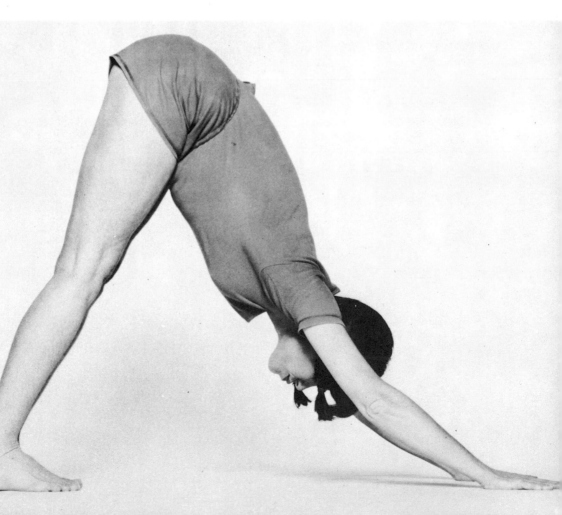

24a

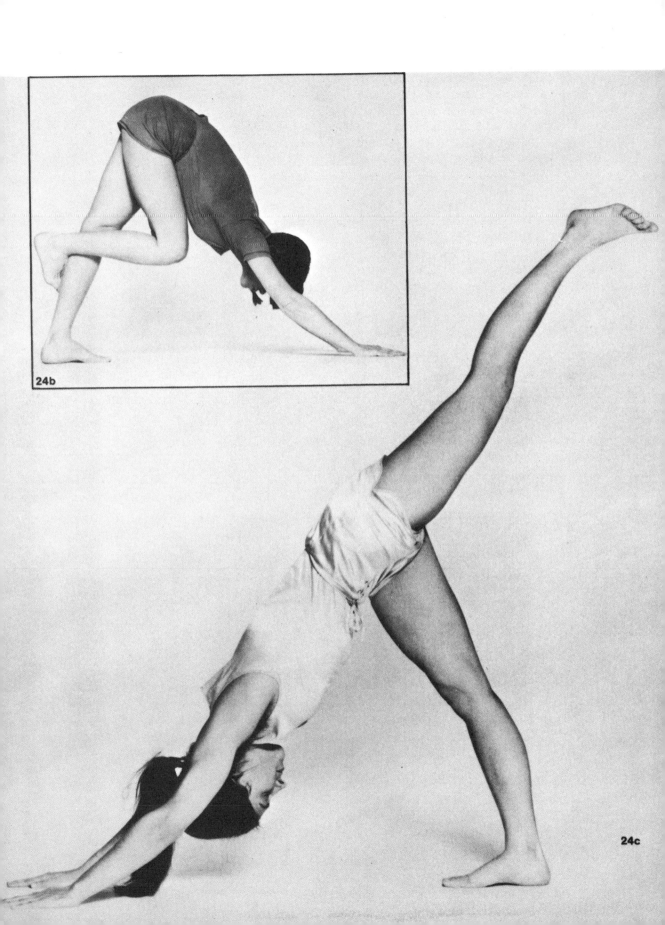

24b

24c

## Movement 25: The tailor position

Sit on the floor with your legs stretched straight out in front of you. Bend your knees and at the same time bring the soles of your feet together. Grip your feet and bring them as close to your groin as possible. Widen your thighs and lower your knees as far as you can on to the floor. Try to sit upright by sitting on the front of your buttock bones and not the back. If this is difficult sit on a cushion with your back against a wall. To help your knees down you may push your thighs with your elbows, but it is better to make progress gradually without doing this. Start with 1 minute and increase to 5 or 10 minutes. You can also lift your thighs slightly and drop them in rhythm, building up momentum.

Soles of feet together. Draw feet to groin. Trunk straight and relaxed. Sit lightly on the front of buttock bones. Take knees to the floor as much as possible.

The most common fault in this sitting position is the trunk falling back because you are not sitting on the front of the buttock bones.

25

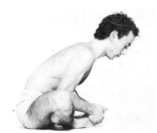

26a

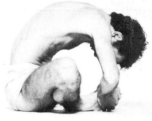

26b

## Movement 26: Bending pelvis and trunk forward in the tailor position

When you can sit upright with relative ease and your knees are well lowered to the floor, try to bend your pelvis and trunk forward from your buttock bones (**26a**). The most common mistake (**26b**) is to overbend the trunk and not move from the buttocks, as can be seen in the photographs. There is a correct and incorrect way of bending, even if the movement is limited.

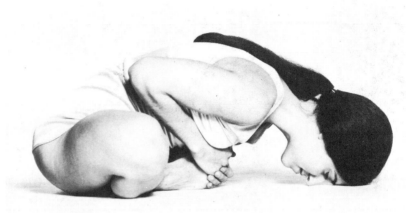

26c

### Final position (26c)

Go forward with pelvis and trunk. Lever from buttock bones. Lower abdomen on to feet. Minimum bending of trunk.

### Variation (26d,e)

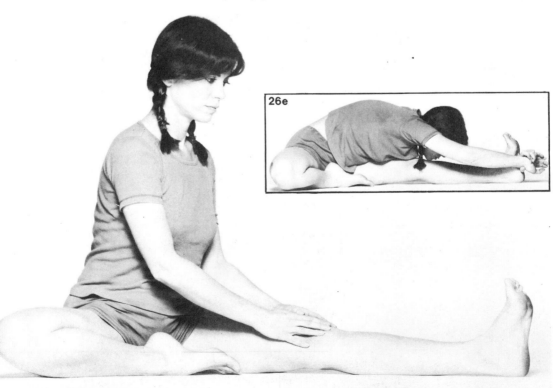

26e

26d

### Movement 27: Bending pelvis and trunk on to extended legs

Do not attempt the following movement until you are able to bend your pelvis and trunk forward in the standing position (Movement 12, page 69).

If that position is easy, try this:

Sit on the floor with your legs stretched out in front of you. Straighten your knees and do not point your toes but rather extend your heels. Your trunk should be straight and relaxed, sitting on the front of your buttock bones (**27a**).

Reach forward, with your trunk straight, and grip your feet. Now, from your buttock bones, lever your pelvis and trunk forward. Bring your lower abdomen and chest on to your thighs. Finally bring your face on to your knees (**27b**).

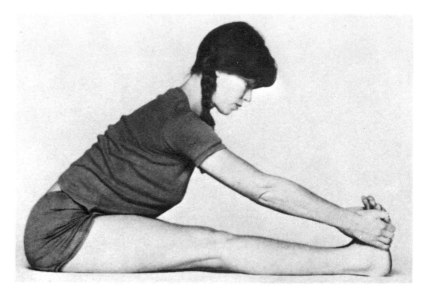

**27a** Knees together and straight. Heels extended. Lever pelvis and trunk from buttock bones.

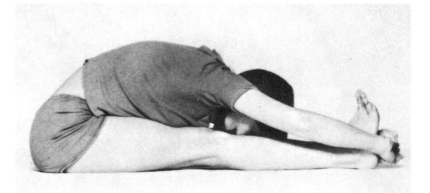

**27b** Abdomen and chest on thighs, face on knees.

When this movement can be done easily and your hamstrings are lengthened and relaxed, try the following variations:

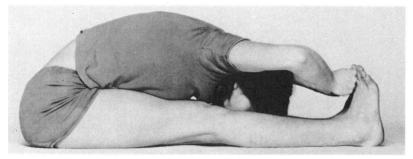

**27c** Gripping big toes.

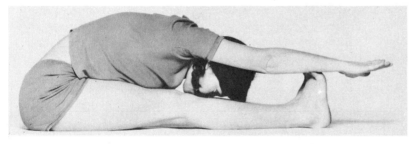

**27d** Arms extended forward.

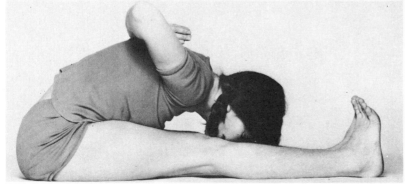

**27e** Hands joined behind back, palm to palm.

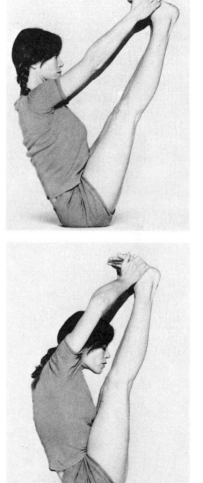

**27f,g** Balancing on buttocks.

95

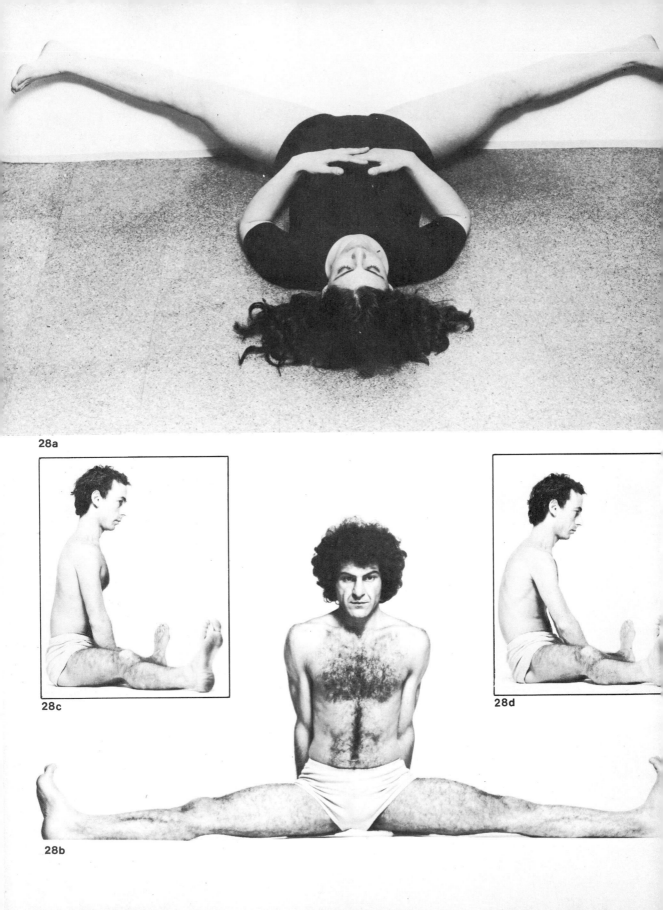

28a

28c

28d

28b

## Movement 28: Sitting with feet as wide apart as possible

To spread your legs as wide as possible, begin by lying on your back, buttocks against a wall, forming an L. Slowly spread your legs apart as far as they will go. Keep your knees extended but not tight. Do not point your toes (**28a**). This simple movement lengthens and relaxes your inner thigh muscles, the adductors.

Your back is supported and safe, but, since these thigh muscles are very large, be careful at first how long you stretch them. Stay in the position only as long as it is comfortable.

When this exercise becomes easy, sit on the floor with your legs extended in front of you. Now spread them apart as far as possible. Make sure your knees are extended. Turn your feet towards your knees, extending your heels. This movement involves first of all sitting upright, trunk straight, with your weight on the front part of your buttock bones. If this is difficult use a cushion with your back on a wall or push backwards with your arms to lift lightly (**28b**).

The most common failing in carrying out this movement is not lifting up the back from the buttocks (**28d**). (**28c**) is correct.

### Final position (28e)

Legs as far apart as possible. Feet pointing towards knees. Weight on the front of buttocks. Trunk and pelvis straight.

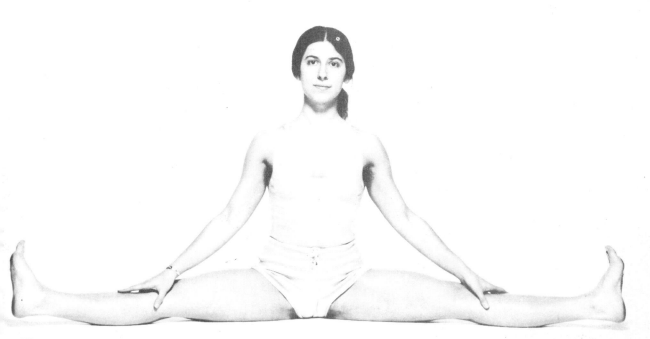

**28e**

## Movement 29: Bending trunk and pelvis forward with legs apart

Before attempting the next position you should be able to sit in the last position with ease and have practised a similar standing position (Movement 14, page 74).

Bend your trunk and pelvis forward together, using your buttock bones as the point of leverage, and bring your abdomen forward. Avoid overbending your back. Even if your movement is limited you can see from the photographs the correct (**29a**) and incorrect (**29b**) leverage.

Make sure your knees are fully extended and your feet point towards your knees, extending your heels. You can also use rhythmic movements to gain momentum (**29c-f**). Breathe out as you go down and breathe in as you come up.

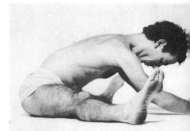

29a

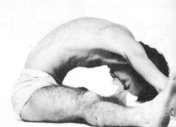

29b

### Final position (29g)

Feet spread as wide apart as possible. Knees fully extended. Feet point to knees. Lever pelvis and trunk from buttocks. Abdomen goes down towards the floor.

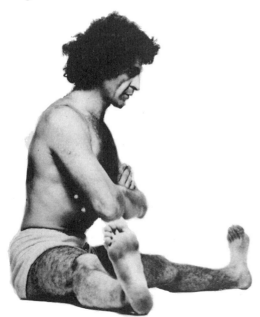
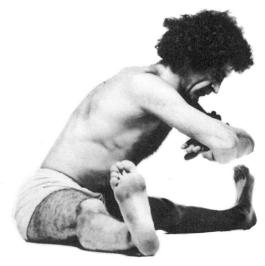

29g

29c

29d

If this is reasonably easy, try these variations (**29h,i**):

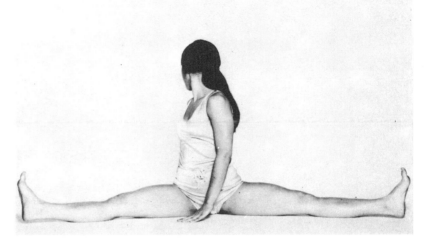

**29h** Twist trunk to look behind your back, left and right sides.

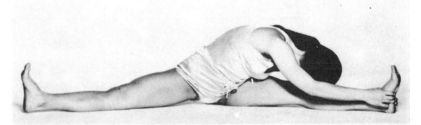

**29i** Bend to each side alternately.

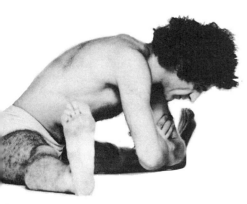

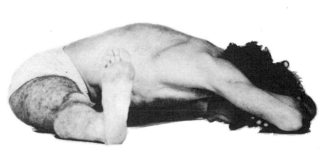

29e

29f

**Movement 30: Sitting between your feet**

Before you can sit between your feet, you should be able to sit on them. Begin sitting on them until it is not difficult to do so for 3 to 5 minutes. Then, each time you do the exercise and have been sitting for a few minutes, draw your feet apart in gradual stages until eventually your buttocks rest on the floor. Make sure that your toes turn slightly inwards and your heels outwards (**30a**).

If sitting between your feet with your knees together is too difficult, try sitting on a cushion.

Try these arm variations (**30b-d**):

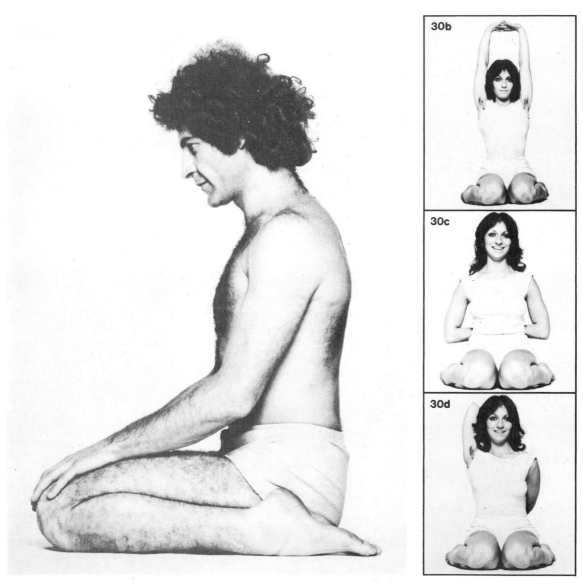

**30a** Sit between feet, buttocks on the floor and knees together. Toes should turn slightly inwards and heels outwards.

## Movement 31: Sitting between your feet and bending your pelvis and trunk forward

After you have become accustomed to sitting between your feet, bend your pelvis and trunk forward from your buttock bones (**31a**). They lift up to begin with but with time and practice your buttocks will eventually remain on the floor. Avoid overbending your back and trunk.

**31a** Lever forward from buttock bones. Abdomen and chest down on to thighs. Try this arm variation (**31b**). Hands behind back, palm to palm.

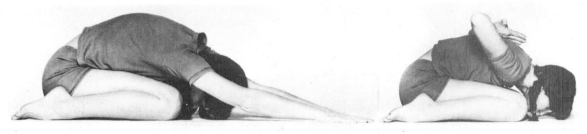

31a

31b

Try these leg variations (**31c-f**):

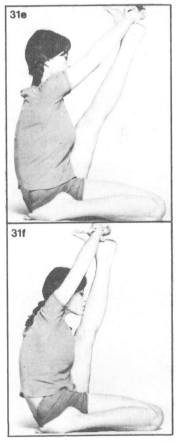

31e

31f

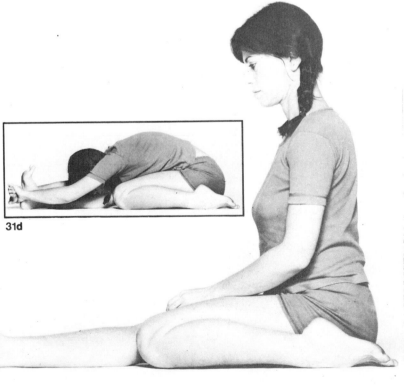

31d

31c

## Movement 32: Sitting between your feet, knees apart

Sitting between your feet, spread your knees as wide as possible, and bring your toes to touch each other behind your buttocks (**32a**). This is a popular Japanese sitting position. When you can do it comfortably, try levering your pelvis and trunk forward on to the ground (**32b**).

32a

32b

## Movement 33: Lengthening and relaxing hamstrings lying down

Lie on your back with your feet together. Bend one knee, bringing it towards your chest. Use your hands to pull your knee in further (**33a**).

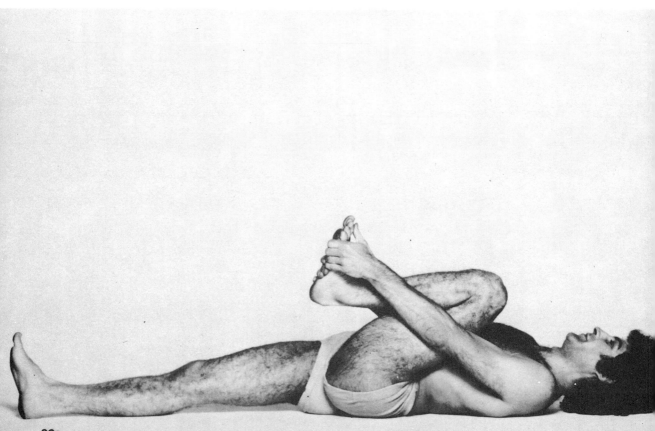

33a

**Stage 1** Next, straighten your knee, if you can. If this is difficult, hold your ankle or lower down, but make sure your knee is fully extended (**33b**).

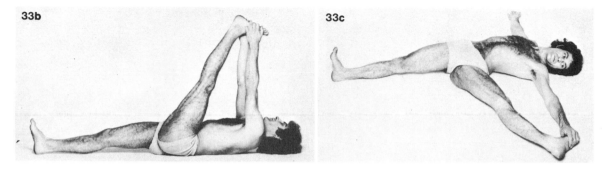

**Stage 2** When the last movement is easy, try this: Take one arm to your side, as in the photograph (**33c**) then take your leg to the side.

**Stage 3** Return to the previous position and then take your leg to the other side (**33d,e**).

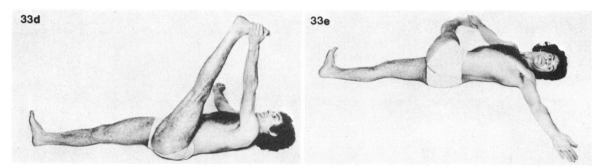

Repeat these movements with the other leg. Treat each stage as a separate movement.

**Stage 4** Now grip both feet and gently pull them towards you (**33f**).

Next, gripping your big toes, widen your feet as much as possible (**33g**).

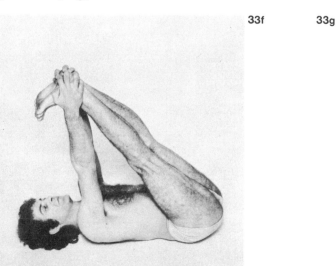
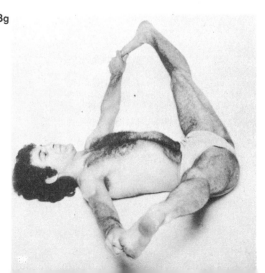

**Stage 5** When you have become proficient in these, try the next movement.
**Movement 34: The splits** Repeat on other side (**34a,b**).

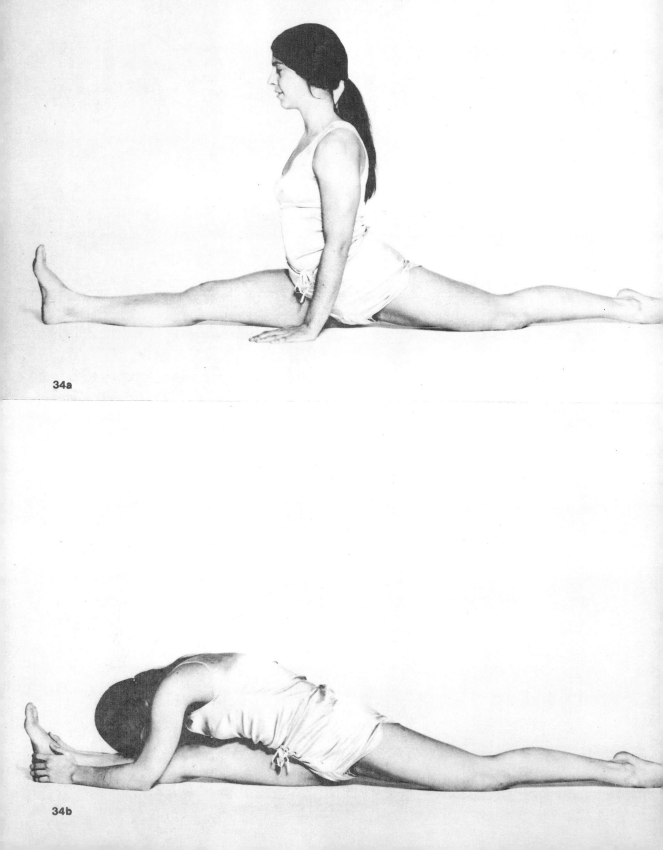

34a

34b

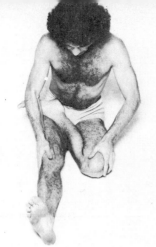

35a

## Movement 35: The lotus position

After your knees have lowered in the tailor position, you may begin to try the lotus position.

Sit with your legs stretched out in front of you, bend one knee, and with your hands bring your ankle on to your thigh. Slowly and cautiously work your bent knee to touch the floor, and then to rest, next to your extended knee, as in the photograph (**35a**). Repeat with the other knee.

When this is reasonably easy, try the full lotus position. Your knees should be as close together as possible and your ankles well up on your thighs (**35b**).

Now lever your pelvis and trunk forward to the floor (**35c**).

Try these variations (**35d-f**).

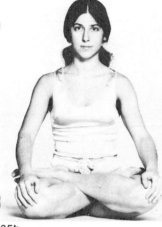

35b

35c

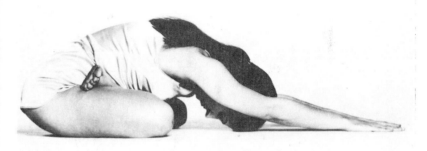

35f

35d

35e

All the movements so far have dealt with forward bending of your pelvis and trunk. The next two movements deal with the extension of your pelvis and trunk.

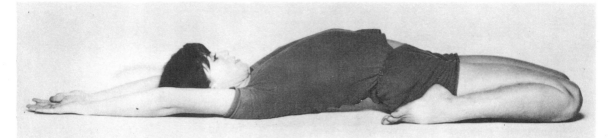

36a

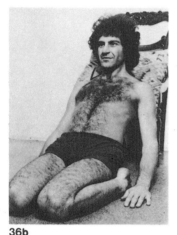

36b

**Movement 36: Lying back between your feet, knees together**
Sit between your feet; if you cannot, sit on a cushion. Slowly lean back on to your elbows and then on to your back (**36a**). Stop the movement if you feel any pain in your lower back. Your hip joints are larger and stronger than your lower back joints; therefore, if your hips are tight, the strain falls on the lower back.

Try to tilt your pelvis up as much as possible by moving your buttock bones towards your knees and the tops of your hip bones towards the ground. The less your trunk is curved the better. To work your body gradually into this position, place a chair against a wall. Put a cushion on the edge of the chair, and slowly lean back against it (**36b**).

Increase your angle of extending back in stages.

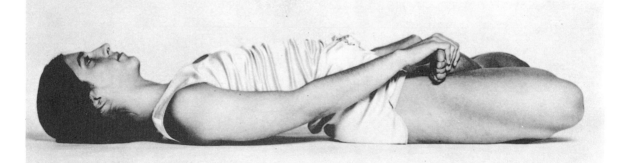

37

**Movement 37: Lying back in lotus**
Sit in the lotus position and lean back on to your elbows. Slowly lower your back on to the floor.

Be sure to stop the moment you feel any pain in your lower back. The aim is to extend your hip joints and lengthen your front thigh muscles, without overbending your backbone and trunk.

Of the twenty-six movements given in this section, the most important can be reduced to these ten:

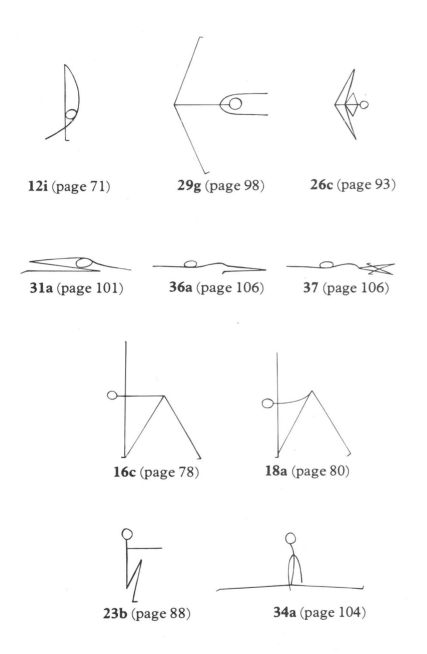

**12i** (page 71)        **29g** (page 98)        **26c** (page 93)

**31a** (page 101)        **36a** (page 106)        **37** (page 106)

**16c** (page 78)        **18a** (page 80)

**23b** (page 88)        **34a** (page 104)

If these ten positions can be done effortlessly, then your ankles, knees and hip joints are truly flexible. The muscles operating them are able to lengthen and shorten fully. Your legs, thighs and buttocks will be at their optimum.

# Rotating trunk

Your backbone is capable of rotation, and so too, therefore, is your trunk. These positions promote that ability.

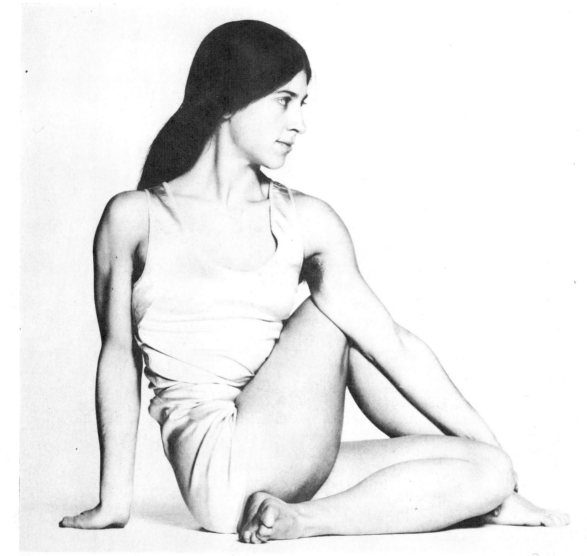

38

**Movement 38: Twist One**
Sit with your knees straight and feet together. Bring one foot over the opposite thigh and place it on the floor. Bend your other knee and slide your foot next to your buttock. Turn your trunk and extend your arm over your upright knee; your arm should be straight, gripping your foot. Rest your other hand on the floor and rotate your trunk, especially between your shoulderblades. Your head can turn to the front or back. Repeat on the opposite side.

### Movement 39: Twist Two

Sit on the floor with your legs stretched out in front of you. Bend one knee and place your foot on the floor. Turn your trunk about 90 degrees, your chest going beyond the bent thigh. Now join your hands, as in the photograph.

To rotate your hips, extend your front hip with your extended leg forward, and your back hip with your bent knee backwards. To rotate your trunk, twist your backbone and shoulders, especially the area between your shoulderblades.

39

### Movement 40: Twist Three

Lie on your front with your hands together under your head. Turn your face to the left, resting it comfortably on your hands. Bend your knees at right angles. Then take both feet to the right very slowly. Hold for 10 seconds and then straighten your legs. Do this very slowly, five times. Repeat on the right with your head turned to the right.

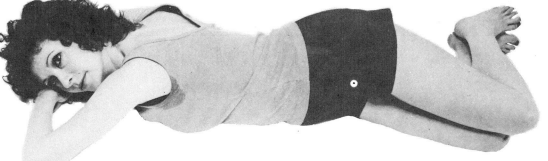

40

Besides these three exercises, you can rotate your trunk in any of these sitting positions:

**1** Sitting with your legs stretched in front of you.
**2** Sitting on your heels.
**3** Sitting with your legs as far apart as possible.
**4** Sitting in the lotus position.

Practice of these promotes your body's ability to rotate to the left and right with ease.

# Bending back or extending trunk

When standing you are able to bend forward far more than you can bend backwards. However, your trunk itself is more capable of backward than forward bending.

Forward bending of your body is allowed by the movement of your hip joints, aided by the movement of your vertebrae, while in backward bending the emphasis is the other way round. You bend back through the movements of your vertebrae aided by those of your hips. Once your trunk has become stiff, for whatever reason, it is not easy to regain flexibility. But it can be done. Before you try to extend your trunk you should be able to extend your hip joints and your shoulder joints – two positions which should be easy (Movement 36 page 106 and Movement 5a page 64).

**Movement 41: Backward bending on table**
Begin this way. Place a mat or a thick folded blanket on a solid table against a wall. The table should not be too wide. Lie on the table on your back with your buttocks against the wall, your knees bent and your feet on the wall. This ensures that your lower back lies firmly on the table. Lie so that your head just hangs over the edge of the table (see page 63).

Allow your head to hang freely with your lower jaw closed against your upper jaw. Do not open your mouth, or you will not get the proper throat stretch. Always make sure your lower back does not lift up and curve. All the front muscles of the top half of your body are being lengthened and relaxed, helped by gravity, and without resistance, strain or stress on your lower back.

After your head is able to remain comfortably in this position for a few minutes, the next stage is to take your arms overhead with fingers interlocked (**41a,b**). Then jut your head further out over the edge of the table, a little at a time, stage by stage. Stay in each stage for as long as is comfortable until you build up to an easy 5 minutes.

This is the only safe way to extend your backbone and stretch the front muscles of your body.

You will realize how vital this exercise is when you think how much of your day you spend hunched forward and how much of your life you have spent like that. Continually hunched up, your front muscles shorten and lose their ability to lengthen. The only way to bring life to your frontal body muscle groups is passively to lengthen them in order to release their tension and prolonged contraction. It is safe to do these exercises if you proceed with caution and care. Aim at gradual progress.

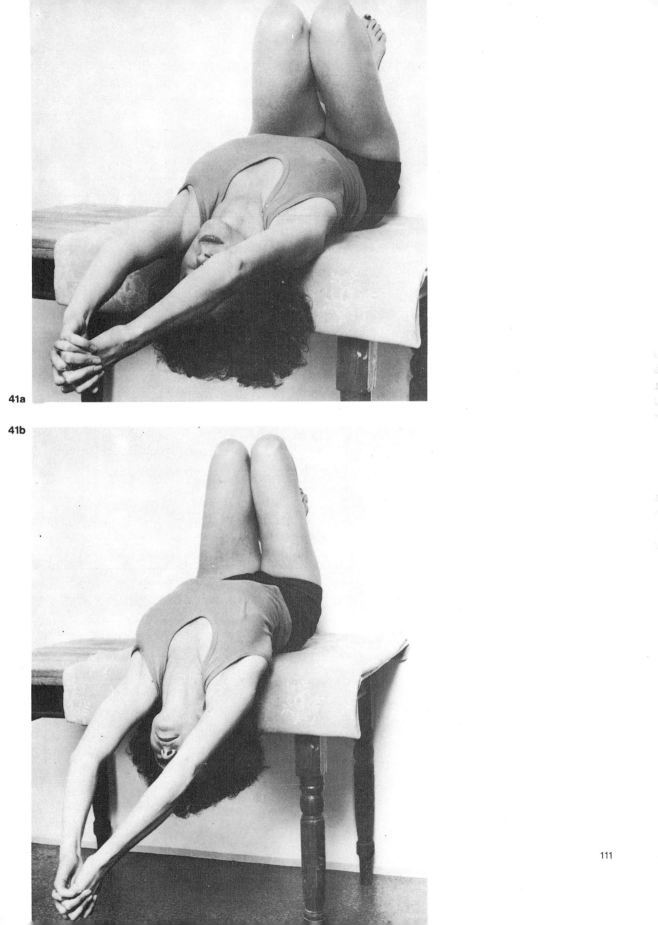

**41a**

**41b**

111

## Movement 42: Backward bending, sitting on heels

In the next movement to promote the flexibility of your trunk, start by sitting on your feet about 3 feet from a wall. Without leaning back, lift your arms overhead, bend your trunk in the middle and touch the wall behind you. Exhale as you extend back and inhale as you come down. Do this slowly. Hold it for 15 seconds. Repeat the movement ten times.

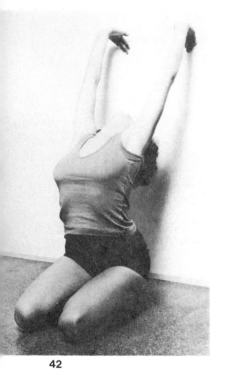

42

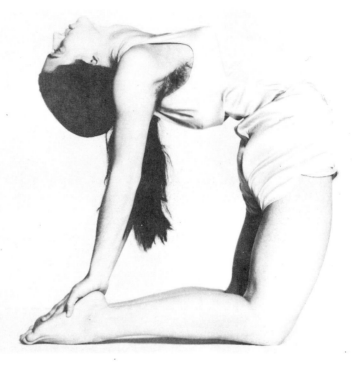

43

## Movement 43: The camel position

Kneel on the floor, your thighs and feet together. Rest your hands on your hips, stretch your thighs and extend your trunk backwards. Now place your palms on your heels. Make sure that your thighs are perpendicular to the floor or, better, slightly forward.

## Movement 44: The crab position

Lie on the floor. Bend and raise your elbows over your head and place your palms under your shoulders. Your fingers should point towards your feet. Bend your knees and bring your feet close to your buttocks. Breathe out and raise your trunk, resting your head on the floor. Rest a few seconds, then stretch your arms from your shoulders until your elbows are straightened, at the same time pulling your thighs up. Relax your head and neck and lift up your abdomen as high as possible (**44a**).

When this is easy, try extending your legs (**44b**).

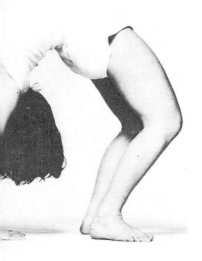

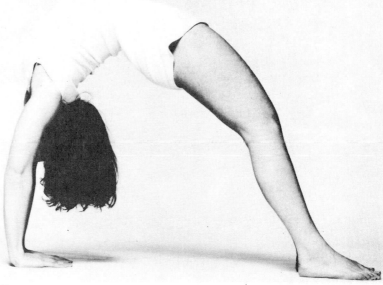

44a

44b

### The cobra and dog positions
In these positions you bend your trunk against the force of gravity. They should be tried only when your backbone is reasonably flexible.

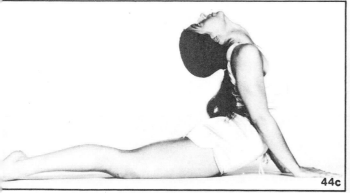

44c

### The cobra position (44c)
Thighs, hands and feet in contact with the floor.

### The dog position (44d)
Only the back of feet and hands in contact with floor.

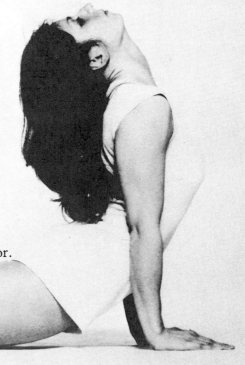

44d

# Strengthening abdominal muscles

In these three exercises, the muscles of your abdomen act as fixators. They fix your pelvis to your trunk so that the muscles raising your legs have a firm base from which to pull. They are practised to strengthen and tone your abdominal muscles.

### Movement 45: The boat position
Sit with knees straight and together. Lean back, raising your legs above the level of your head, with your arms parallel to the floor. Hold for 10 seconds and build up to about 30.

### Movement 46: The second boat position
Now try a similar movement, but placing your hands behind your head. Your face and feet should be about the same height off the floor. Again hold for 10 seconds and build up to 30.

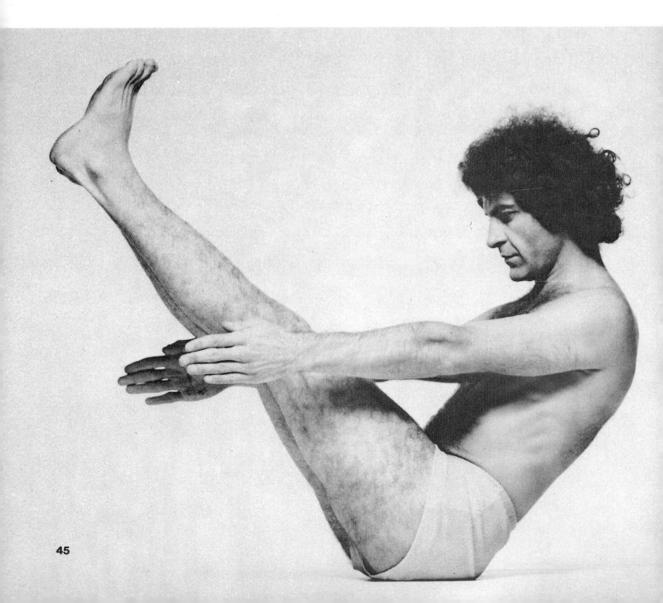

## Movement 47

Lie on your back with arms overhead. Now raise both your feet to the vertical (**47a**). Hold this for half a minute, lower your legs to about 60 degrees (**47b**), hold for 15 seconds, next lower to 15 degrees (**47c**), hold for 15 seconds. Then place your feet on the floor and rest.

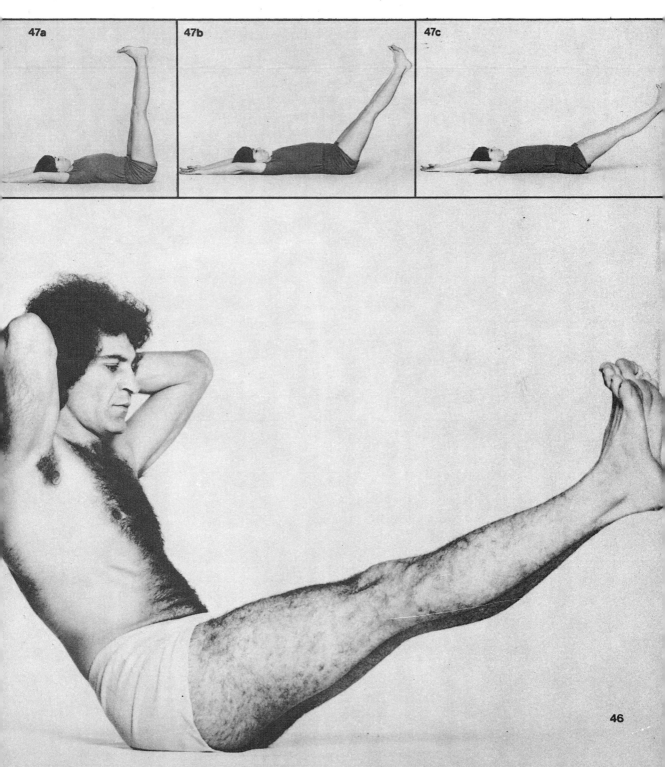

**46**

# Hands

Your hands are important to you from the day you are born. One of your first movements is an involuntary grasp. Later you make more deliberate grabs and after only a few months your eyes are able to focus on your hands. Then you bring them together and start to play. It is not long before you begin to grasp everything within reach.

Your hands are more specialized than those of any animal. Indeed, the really important change that came with standing erect was the freeing of our arms and hands from the job of support and locomotion. They were then able to develop their own skills, making possible the enormous versatility of 'man the toolmaker'. It is not surprising that of the brain tissue that controls your body's movements, a greater proportion is devoted to the movements of your hands than to any other mechanical function.

Yet hands are even more than tools. The handshake symbolizes greeting, the handclasp mutual goodwill.

Twenty-seven bones and twenty muscles give each hand its diversity in action. There are eight small wrist bones in two rows. Your two forearm bones articulate with the first of these rows. The structure of the joints allows your hand to make movements at your wrist independent of those at your elbow.

Flexion and extension of your wrist and abduction and adduction of your hand are produced by the ulnar and radial flexors and extensors, the ulnar flexor and extensor causing adduction while the radial flexor and extensor cause abduction; the flexors and extensors of your fingers are also enlisted for greater power. In each hand, up to your knuckles, five bones, the metacarpals, stretch across your palm and are joined to your fingers and thumbs. There are three bones in each finger and two in the thumb. The bones of your fingers are jointed to allow separate movement of each one.

Although the design and construction of your hand explain its overall flexibility, it is your thumb that provides the real strength of your hand. Without the special grasp of your thumb, most of the power of your hand would be lost. The saddle-shaped bone across the hinge at your thumb joint adds another axis of movement, allowing it to move forward and from side to side, so that thumb and fingers together open up an enormous range of manipulations.

Embedded in your forearms are most of the muscles that control the movements of your hands. If you clench your fist, you can feel some of these muscles contracting. Tendons run across your wrist from your hand to the muscles of your forearm that control the actions of your fingers. The tone of these twelve muscles ensures their maximum flexibility of motion.

Training your hands to carry out all the work they are capable of achieves the co-ordination of the highly complex system of muscles and joints and the nerves that connect every part of your hand to your brain. This involves making your hands thoroughly flexible. There appears to be no other method than the kind described below of improving that flexibility.

We have pointed out earlier that antagonistic muscles can be lengthened and rested in extreme movements by outside forces. Use the force of the opposite hand as that outside force to extend, bend and rotate all the joints of your hands.

## Movements to promote the flexibility of your hands

Each finger can bend and extend at three different joints and your thumbs at two joints.

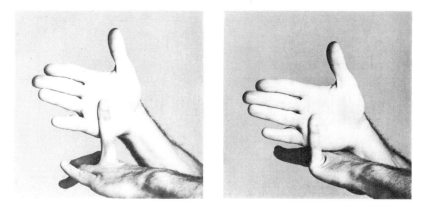

**1a,b** Press back each finger until it is nearly at right angles to your palm.

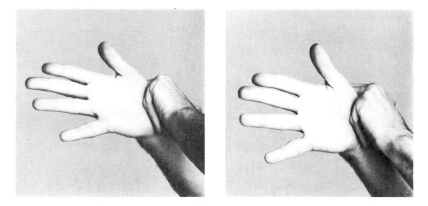

**2a,b** Flex the root joint of each finger fully. Your joints may make a cracking sound. This is good.

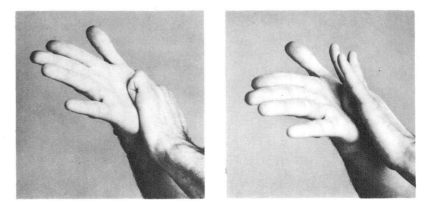

**3a,b** Bend the middle joints of each finger as much as possible.

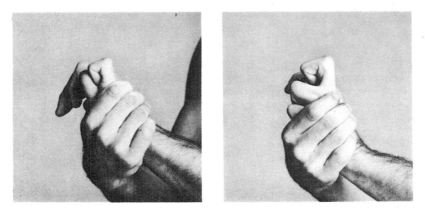

**4a,b** Bend the top finger joints as much as possible.

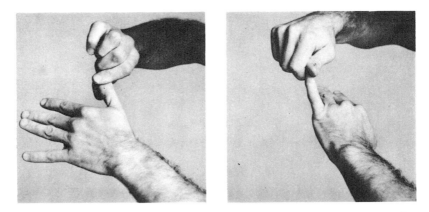

**5a,b** Rotate all your fingers and thumbs, first one way, then the other.

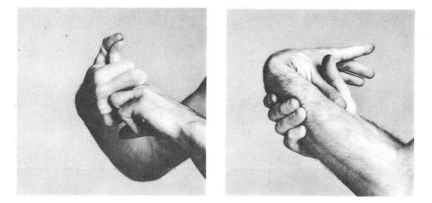

**6a** Bend all your top finger joints backwards.
**6b** Press your thumb down towards your lower arm.

These movements assist the flexibility of all twenty-eight joints of your fingers and thumbs.

Now try deep thumb pressure all over the palm of each hand, and with your fingers knead the fleshy shank of each thumb. Then thoroughly knead the web between your thumb and index finger. Finally, shake both your hands by flicking your wrists.

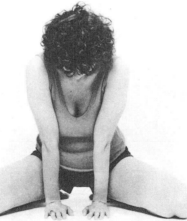

# Wrists

**Movements to promote the flexibility of your wrists**
The ability to bend your wrists at a perfect right angle is a sign of relaxed and harmonious muscles acting on those joints. If you cannot do this, sit on your feet, with knees apart, and place your hands in front of you on the floor. Fingers should be pointed upwards, as in the photograph. Now lever your body forward until your arm and hand are at right angles. Stay in this position for as long as is comfortable. Now try the reverse, your wrist bending the other way.

These two movements promote the flexibility of your wrists and lengthen and relax all the muscles operating them.

# *Feet*

Your foot is an architectural marvel – an engineering masterpiece. It has twenty-six bones, nineteen muscles, around a hundred ligaments, and an intricate network of tendons, which act as guy ropes or slings for the arches. When these components are perfectly balanced, the foot can handle almost any amount of work.

However, even a minute deviation from normal can cause adjustments that will eventually produce injury either to the foot or its supporting muscles and tendons, and even in the knees, hips and lower back. Most muscle tears, pulls and strains occur because of lack of flexibility, which is fundamentally the imbalance of opposing muscle action. The balanced conditioning of individual muscle groups not only protects the foot against injury, but also improves its performance and the performance of your entire body.

To support the weight of your body, as well as permitting free and adaptable movement, demands a very strong and flexible mechanism. This is provided by the arch-like structures of your feet, a physical engineering feature exclusive to humans. You do not stand flat on your feet; you stand on two heels and two soles.

**Movements to promote the flexibility of your feet**
A brief survey of the foot will help you to understand its workings, as the bones of your foot are arranged in a series of arches.

Your foot is supported at the front by the under surfaces of your toes and the round parts of the bones behind your toes (the ball of your foot), and at the back by your heel bone. These supports form the pillars of the long arch of your foot. It is raised off the ground on its inner side. The weight of your body is transmitted from the highest part of the arch to your front foot and heel.

All the bones are kept in place by ligaments, supported by tendons (leaders) of muscles from your leg, which form strong unyielding cords that hold your foot steady and firm. They are assisted by muscles on the side of your foot.

Place both your feet closely together. You will notice that the two inside curves of your feet form a complete dome. Each foot forms a half-dome. The bones from the outer side to the inner side form this curve. It is known as the transverse arch, or small arch, of the foot.

The preservation of the long and short arches is essential to healthy, well-balanced feet. If they collapse, flat or splayed feet are the result.

Examine the shape of your foot. Your big toe should be in line with the inner margin of your foot (that is, pointed straight forward) and the rest of the toes straight, lying with the whole of their under surfaces in contact with the floor.

Your feet should be soft and supple, with the full range of movements in their various joints, particularly the joints joining your toes to your foot bones.

Test the mobility of your feet:

**1** Place your feet on the ground and try to spread out your toes. Bring your big toes inwards until they are in a straight line with the inner borders of your feet.

**2** Bring your toes together – that is, the four outer toes of each foot should be brought inwards towards your big toes.

**3** With your heels resting on the floor and the front of your feet raised, bend your toes upwards and downwards, noting how far you can make each movement.

**4** With your feet on the floor, raise your heels, that is, stand on tiptoe, so that all five toes of each foot are at right angles to the rest of your foot.

**5** Place your feet on the floor, keeping your toes flat and your heels steady. Raise the inner sides of your feet while drawing your toes backwards towards your heels. (The toes should be pressed down as in tapping, not curled as in grasping.) This movement brings into action the small muscles which support your arches. If it is done properly, the balls of your feet are slightly raised and supported.

If all these movements are free, your feet are efficient and relaxed. If not, action should be taken to improve them. This will involve:

**1** Foot care, that is, the correct stockings or socks and footwear.

**2** Massage (see Chapter 4).

**3** Movements to improve flexibility.

**Fitting footwear**

The feet of stockings or socks must be long enough for your toes to lie flat, otherwise your toes will be curled up, leading to corns above and below your toes and calluses under the pads of your feet.

Shoes should be long enough to allow your toes to lie flat, and wide enough to allow them to spread. Most important, the inner side, which is in contact with the big toe, should be straight and not pointed towards the middle of the toes. A shoe with a wide and rounded toe is preferable to one with a sharply pointed toe.

The flatter the heels of your shoes the better. Shoes with high heels tend to slide your feet too far forward, causing the muscles in your lower back to readjust. This leads to backache and fatigued feet because the weight of your body cannot be sufficiently supported on such a small base.

Shoes that prevent your feet sliding forward (those with a slight built-in arch), with enough room to allow your toes to lie straight, and with flat heels, capable of sustaining the weight of your body, are more suitable. In pregnancy, when body-weight is rapidly increased, foot comfort is essential.

**Supple feet**
Try and improve the contours of your feet if they have lost their shapeliness. Some simple ways of doing this are shown in the photographs below.

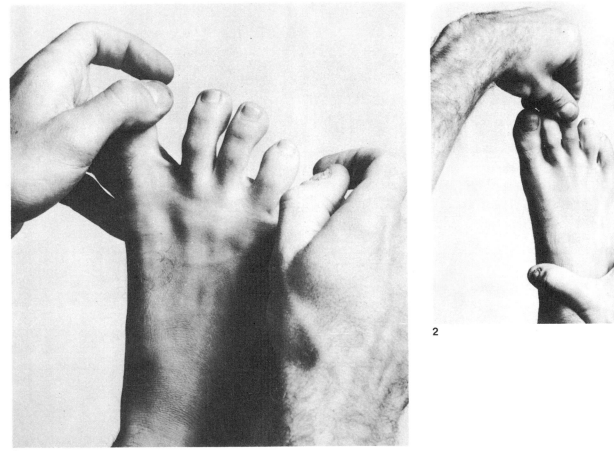

1

2

**1** Spread your toes by separating your big toe from your little toe.
**2** Grasp each toe between your fingers and thumb and pull outwards in the direction of its long axis (traction).

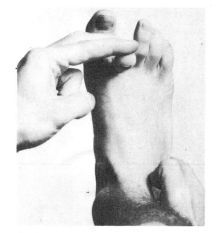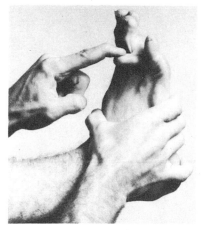

**3a,b** Extend each toe upwards.

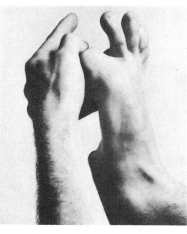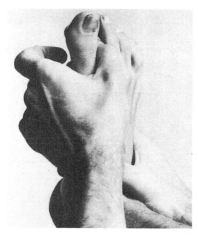

**4a,b** Bend each toe forwards.

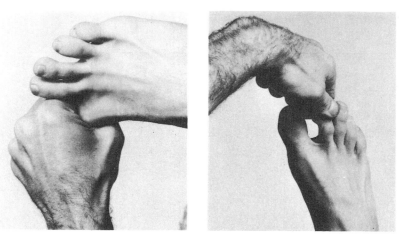

**5a,b** Twist each toe to the left and right.

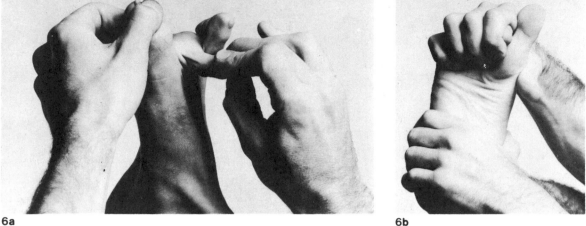

**6a**

**6b**

**6a** 'Scissor' all your toes, one forward and one backward at a time.

**6b** With a forward flick of your wrist, bend and 'crack' your toes.

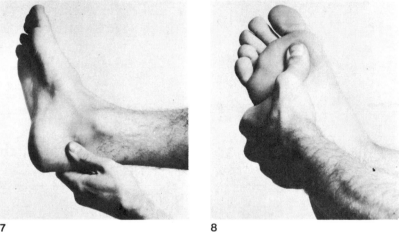

**7**

**8**

**7** Pinch and massage your achilles tendon up and down.

**8** Next, turn the sole of your foot up. Squeeze, roll, knead, and mould it. Place your thumbs on the forepart and 'remould' it into shape. Manipulate it in every direction to enable the various bones to move freely and the whole foot to become soft and supple.

# 13 Balance

The force of gravity pulls your body, like all objects, down towards the centre of the earth. And the only forces you have with which to resist this pull are the obvious force of muscle action and the subtle force of will. At all times, whether you are conscious of it or not, you are challenged by gravity and respond to it through muscle action and will.

These inverted balancing positions emphasize and focus your attention on the basic relationship between your body and gravity. In them you will experience the sensation of weight and the tremendous effort required of your body to balance itself. In your normal upright position, due to familiarity and adjustment, you have mostly become unaware of these factors.

If your body feels heavy, clumsy, floppy or a drag, it indicates that its basic relationship to gravity is out of balance. Mastering these balancing positions brings lightness and ease to your body in your everyday activities. Your body's ability to neutralize gravity automatically improves. The opposite of gravity is grace.

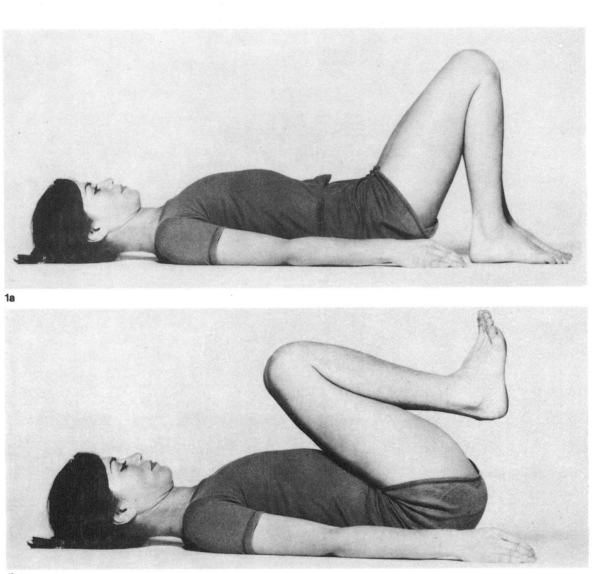

1a

1b

## *Neck-shoulder balance*

Lie flat on your back with your chin in and your palms on the floor. Bend your knees and bring them towards your head as you lift your trunk. Place your hands on your back, sliding your elbows towards each other for extra support.

Point your knees upwards and then straighten your legs. Extend your trunk and make it as perpendicular to the floor as possible. Stretch the front of your body and legs more than the back. Your knees should face slightly inwards and your feet be relaxed. Avoid pointing your toes or tensing your feet (**1a-e**).

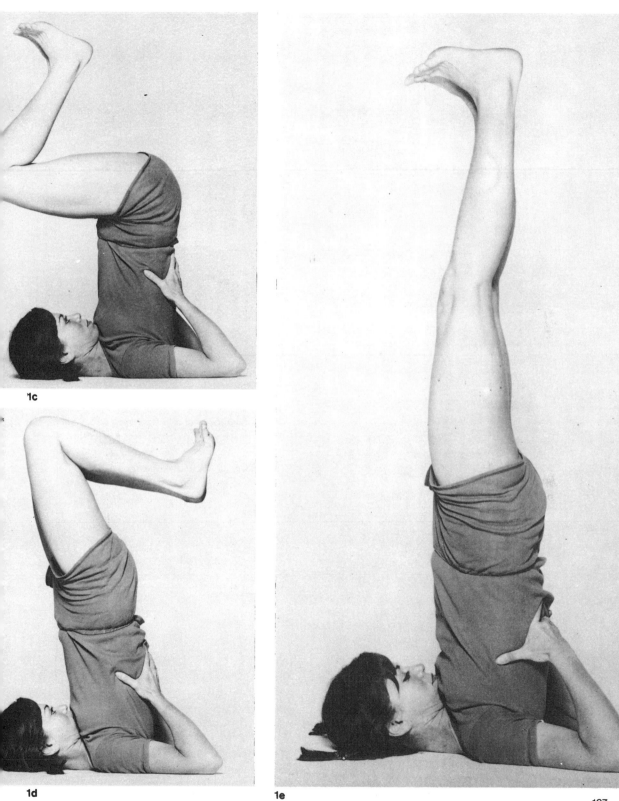

1c

1d

1e

Another way to go into this position is to raise your legs at right angles to your body. Raise your legs further by lifting your trunk from the floor, at the same time placing your hands on your back. Bring your elbows towards each other and straighten up into the full position (**2a-c**). Try to straighten your body and legs by tightening your buttocks and at the same time, stretch your trunk from the bottom of your breastbone to your groin.

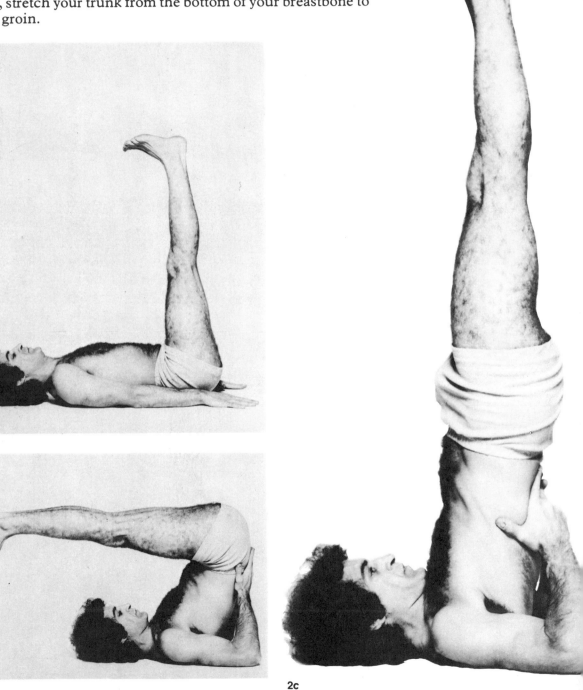

2a

2b

2c

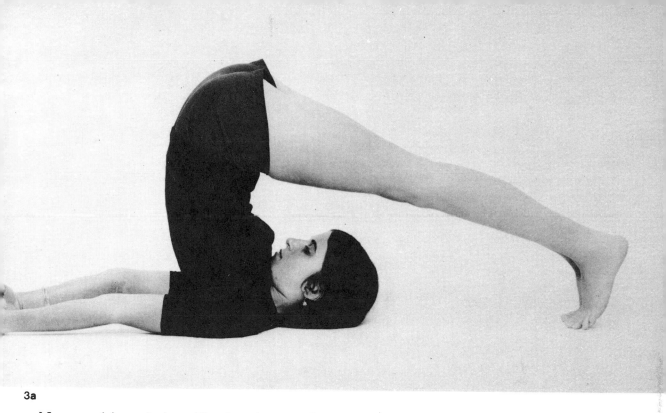

Now try this variation: Slowly take your feet to the ground and, interlocking your fingers, extend your arms backwards (**3a**). This is called the plough position.

The next variation is to bend your knees and place them near your ears (**3b**).

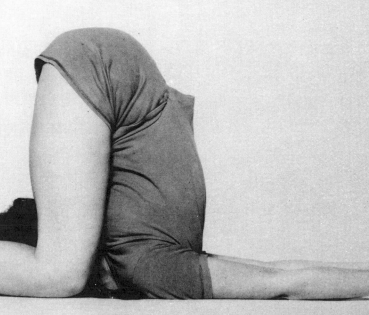

**3b**

Straighten up again and try this: Take your right foot down to the floor and keep it there for about half a minute before returning it to a perpendicular position (3c). Then repeat the movement with the left.

3c

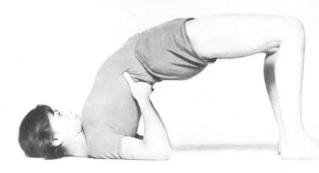

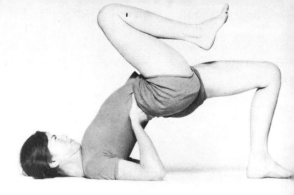

3d

3c

Very slowly bend your knees and, arching your trunk, lower your feet on to the floor about 2 feet apart. Be careful not to place a sudden load on your wrists. Try at first to bend backwards one leg at a time (**3d**).

Now lift up your right knee, and, flexing it, bring it as close as possible to your chest (**3e**). Then straighten the knee, hold for 10 to 15 seconds and repeat on the other side (**3f**). Place both feet on the ground again. With one leg leading, heave your body up again.

Now place your hands on your thighs and balance like this (**3g**).

This entire routine requires only a few minutes. The neck-shoulder balance with your feet together and the plough position should be practised as separate positions. Start with going into the shoulder-neck balance for 30 seconds and add 30 seconds per week until you bring your time up to 5 or 10 minutes. Build up the plough position to 5 minutes.

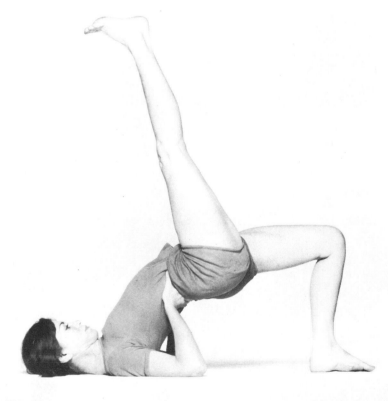

3f

3g

# Head balance

Begin in a corner or against a wall, on a folded blanket. Kneel with your hands linked together on the floor. Your elbows should be apart at shoulder width. Place the crown of your head on the floor, cupping the back of your head with your hands. Keep your neck straight and transfer the weight of your body on to your head and elbows. Walk your legs towards you until your thighs touch your chest. Flex your knees and lift your entire weight on to your head. Now take your knees as high as possible and straighten them out slowly (**4a-d**).

When balancing on your head becomes easy, you may go up with your knees straight, as in the photographs, without using a wall (**4e,f**).

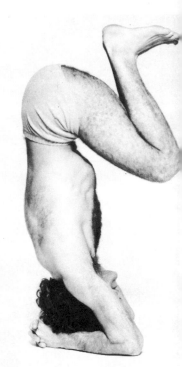

**4b**

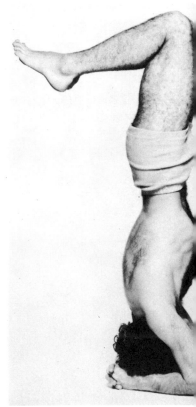

**4c**

**4a**

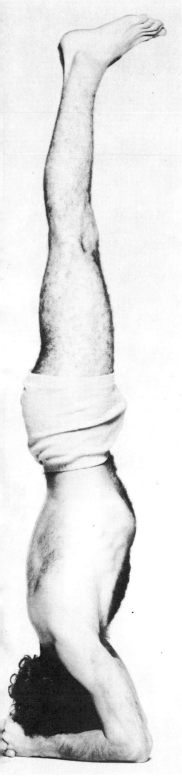

When you are on your head, check out the following:

Lift your shoulderblades gently towards your feet.
Your buttocks should be pulled in and lifted as high as possible towards your heels.
Your pelvis should be level and your abdomen not pushed out.
Avoid over-arching your lower back.
Stretch the back of your legs more than the front, especially from behind your knees to your heels.
Your feet should be easy and not pointed or tense.

Allow ample time for your body to accommodate itself to this inverted position. Start with going into it for, say, 20 seconds for the first week and then add 30 seconds each week until you bring the time up to 5 or 10 minutes. This may require several months. (Sweating in the headstand is a sign to stop.)

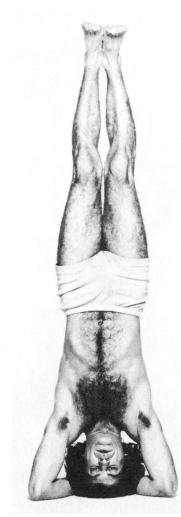

**4e**

**4d**

Only when you are very secure and light on your head, try
these variations (**5a-d**).
You can also vary your arm support (**6a-d**).

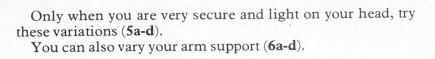

**5a**

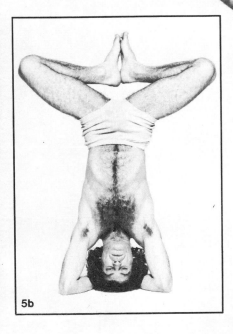

**5b**

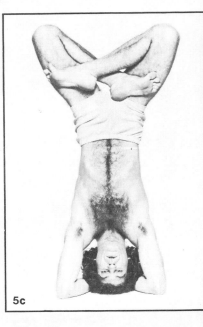

**5c**

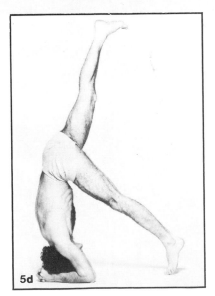

**5d**

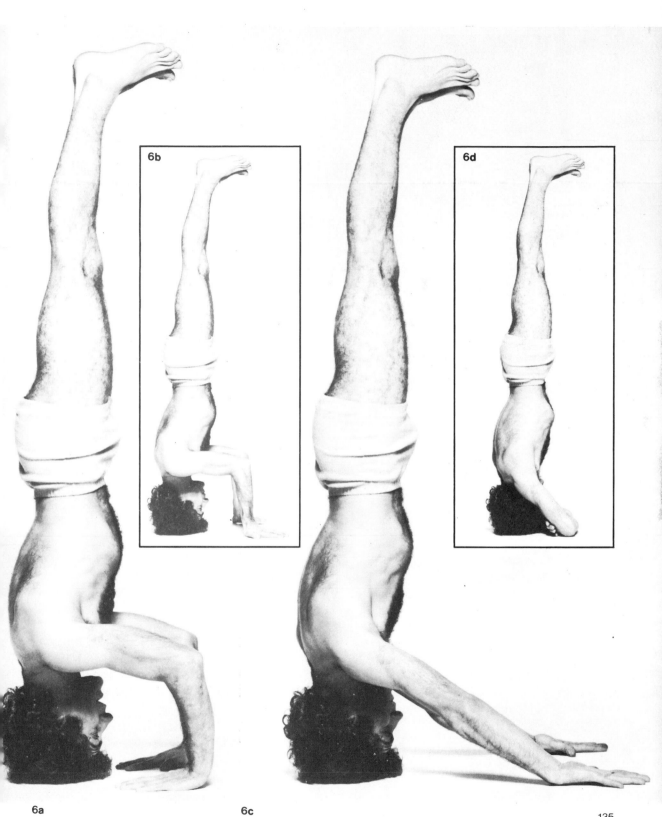

6a

6c

When the neck-shoulder balance and head balance are easy and your body has gained lightness and the ability to resist gravity, you may try these next two balances:

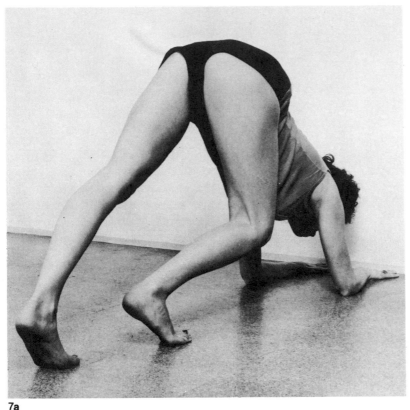

7a

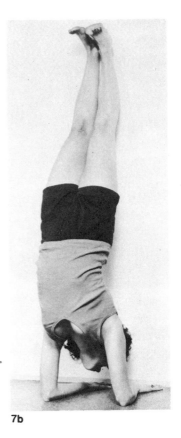

7b

# Elbow balance

Kneel down a few feet from a wall. Place your elbows, forearms and palms on the floor with your fingertips close to the wall. The distance between your elbows should be as wide as your shoulders and your forearm and hands parallel to each other (**7a**). Straighten your legs, and, keeping your head up, swing your left or right leg till it touches the wall, closely followed by your other leg. Once you are up tighten your buttocks and lift them towards your heels. Keep your abdomen in and your lower back curve as shallow as possible. Stretch the back of your legs more than the front. Try to become as tall as possible, edging up the wall with the back of your heels (**7b**).

Stay in this position only as long as is comfortable. Start at 10 seconds and build up to a minute. Practice it until there is no strain on your lower back at all.

The next stage is to take your feet away from the wall without overbending your lower back. After mastering the balance, do the pose in the middle of the room.

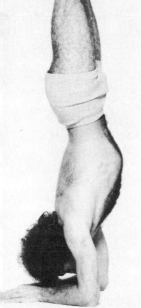

7c

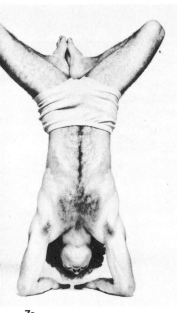

7e

7d

## Final pose without wall (7c)

Elbows shoulder width apart. Forearms parallel to each other. Armpits forward and upper arm vertical. Head and neck firm and relaxed. Lower ribs not protruding forward too far. Buttocks in and up. Back of legs and thighs extended. Feet relaxed and free.

Try these variations when your balance is secure (7d,e).

When balancing, prepare for the sudden change of load. When you step off a pavement that is lower than you expected, you feel a jolt throughout your whole body. This is because you were unprepared for adjusting to the unexpected. In going up into, and even more when coming down from these positions, you must be ready for the shift of load.

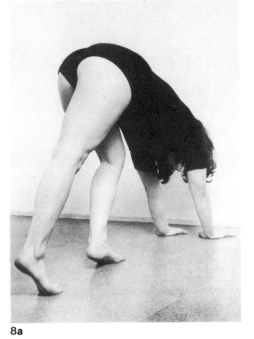

8a

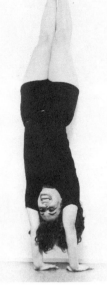

8b

## *Hand balance*

Place your palms about a foot away from a wall. The distance between your palms should be the same as between your shoulders (**8a**). Keeping your elbows fully extended, swing one of your legs up to the wall, followed by the other leg.

Once on the wall, make your body as tall as possible, keeping your abdomen in and your buttocks tight and lifted towards your heels. Stretch the back of your legs, extending your heels on the wall. Keep your feet easy and do not point your toes (**8b**).

Make sure your lower back does not overbend. After you have mastered going up and coming down with ease, try to balance with your feet away from the wall. To start with hold the position for 10 seconds and add 10 seconds per week until you build up to a minute. Then try this position in the middle of the room.

**Final pose (8c)**
Fingers slightly spread and active. Arms parallel and vertical. Armpits forwards. Lower ribs not protruding and body walls parallel. Buttocks in and up. Knees extended. Back thighs and legs extended. Neck firm but relaxed. Head up or down. Feet free.

When you have mastered these four balancing positions, together they should take about 12 minutes (5 in the neck-shoulder balance; 5 in the head balance; 1 in the elbow balance; 1 in the hand balance).

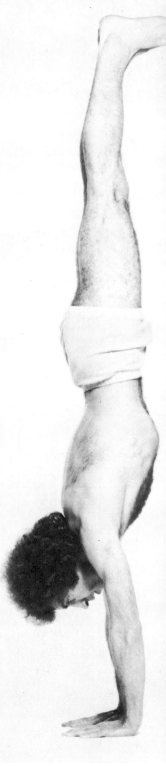

8c

# 14 Resting

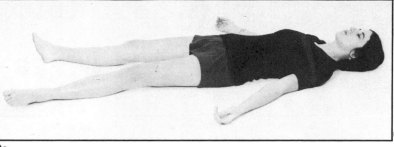

**9a**

Everybody needs to rest. A few moments in a resting position once a day, especially after exertion, will work wonders.

Lie down on a firm surface. If your entire backbone, including your lower back, rests on the floor the position is an effortless one for you( **9a**).

If your lower back does not touch the floor use a cushion and chair (**9b**).

Whichever position you choose, take a few very deep breaths or sigh deeply from way down in your abdomen. With eyes open or closed, become aware of how you feel – not whether you are happy or depressed or bored, but the actual sense of feeling in various parts of your body. This is using the sense of proprioception.

As though it were an exploration into the unknown, feel *from within* all parts of your body. Start with your feet and work upwards to your head, face and finally your eyes. It should be done without effort – a gentle moving awareness of the different parts of your body and then of your body as a whole. The whole secret of successful resting is self-awareness.

Resting is an art, and like any art the more you practise the more efficient you grow. The reward comes only with time. It is the feeling of being wide awake, bright and also at peace.

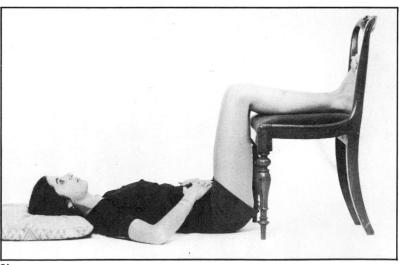

**9b**

# 15 Your movement programme

## Which movements should I start with and in what order?

This depends on which of your joints are stiff. Let us assume that you are rather stiff everywhere, and deal with your body in the following order.

**Your neck** can make only four extreme movements. They are:

**Movement**

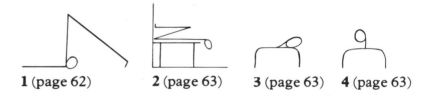

**1** (page 62)      **2** (page 63)    **3** (page 63)   **4** (page 63)

The last two can be done at any time during the day, so put aside time to cultivate the first two. The aim is to make a strenuous, difficult movement into an effortless one.

**Your shoulders** can make five extreme movements. They are:

**1** (page 62)         **5** (page 64)

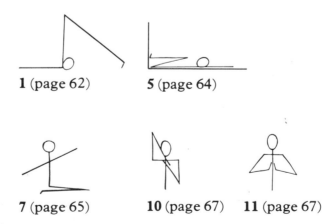

**7** (page 65)    **10** (page 67)   **11** (page 67)

The last three can be done at any time, the first has been included in the neck movements, so add Movement 5 to your programme.

**Your ankles** are capable of two extreme movements:

**23** (page 87)       **24** (page 90)       **30** (page 100)

Add these to your series.

**Your knees** can make these movements.

**30** (page 100)

**12** (page 69)       **25** (page 92)       **35** (page 105)

Add the last three.

**Your hip joints,** which are very large and wide in range, can make these extreme movements:

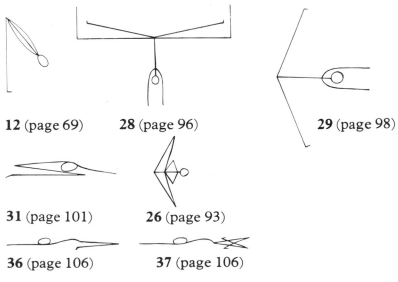

**12** (page 69)       **28** (page 96)                         **29** (page 98)

**31** (page 101)       **26** (page 93)

**36** (page 106)       **37** (page 106)

Add these to your list.

**Your backbone** can bend to the sides, rotate and bend backwards and forwards. Add these extreme movements:

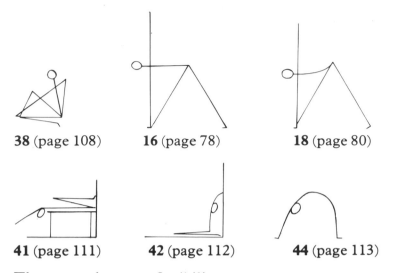

**38** (page 108)     **16** (page 78)     **18** (page 80)

**41** (page 111)     **42** (page 112)     **44** (page 113)

These complete your flexibility programme.

Begin the balancing position with *the neck-shoulder stand* and master that first before going on to *the head stand*. So your final programme, according to your needs, will be something like this:

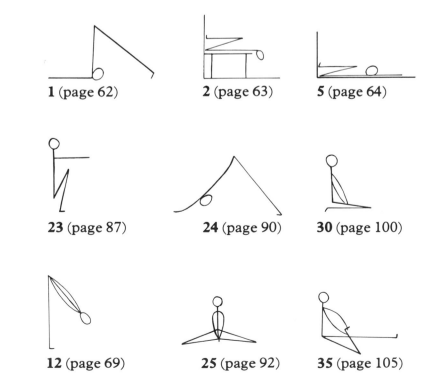

**1** (page 62)     **2** (page 63)     **5** (page 64)

**23** (page 87)     **24** (page 90)     **30** (page 100)

**12** (page 69)     **25** (page 92)     **35** (page 105)

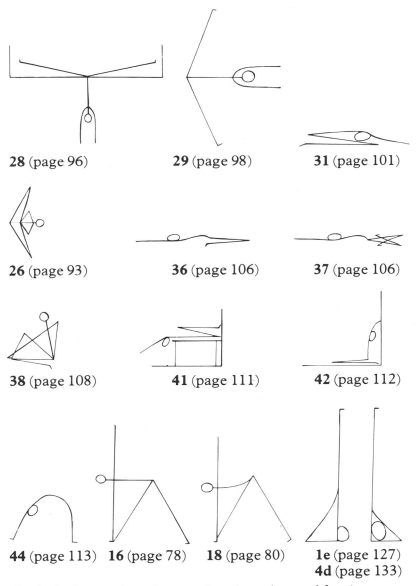

**28** (page 96)          **29** (page 98)          **31** (page 101)

**26** (page 93)          **36** (page 106)          **37** (page 106)

**38** (page 108)          **41** (page 111)          **42** (page 112)

**44** (page 113)   **16** (page 78)   **18** (page 80)   **1e** (page 127)
                                                          **4d** (page 133)

(Include the routines for your hands, wrists and feet.)

No special order is necessary. Vary the movements in any way you find suitable. Become familiar with all of them, but there is no need to do them all in one session. Rest between each position.

At the beginning try to hold the difficult positions for 10 or 15 seconds and repeat three to five times. Increase the time gradually until you can hold them for 1 minute.

It is not advisable to practise after eating, so select a period in the day when your stomach is reasonably empty.

Your body should be warm, so that there is no danger of straining your muscles. For this reason, early morning should be given to self-massage and movements should be done later in the day.

# 16 Practising with two or more

You can do all the movements and positions on your own, but it is often more pleasurable and helpful to practise them with another person or with several. In some of the movements you will find intelligent, gentle assistance by someone else most helpful. If you are assisting someone to further his or her range of movement, never push or use force; with your hands just use your weight gradually, smoothly and gently in the appropriate place. Never use jerky movements, but lever or lean your weight slowly. While gravity or your own body-weight is usually enough to promote the movement in each position, with the' help of another person some movements can be speedily increased in range.

Often the more people (for instance, a whole family) practising these movements together, the more energy and enthusiasm generated. If you decide to work together, it is a good idea to face your partner in all the movements where this is possible, such as most of the standing positions and the head balance. Check out the other's movement, especially noticing when someone is forcing or overbending with strain to get to the final position; also the other's breathing – make sure that the breath is not being held. Always keep looking at the other's face and eyes, which tell a great deal about how he or she is coping with the movement.

In the photographs which follow various ways of promoting movement are shown. They should be attempted only when both partners are familiar with the movements and have cultivated them to a reasonable degree on their own.

When you have both mastered the head balance, do it opposite each other to check the position of the head, neck, shoulders, and so on (1).

1

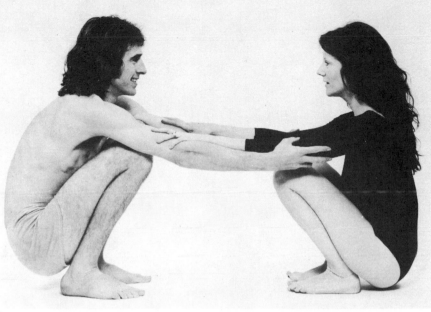

**2**

If squatting on your heels without support is difficult, support each other this way (**2**).

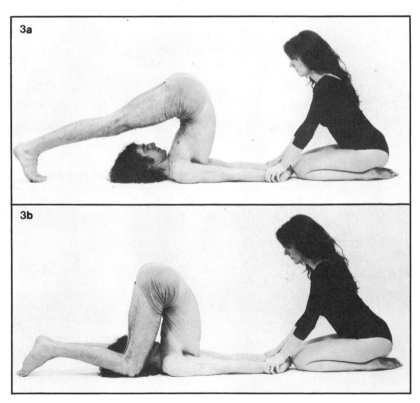

In the plough position, with knees straight or bent, take your partner's arms to the floor by applying pressure gently on the wrists (**3a,b**).

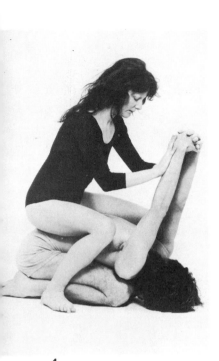

**4**

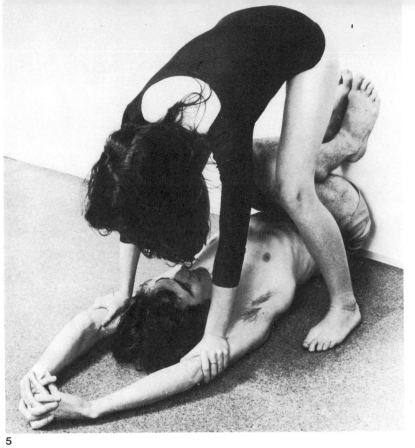

**5**

Sit gently as far back as you can and slowly and gently lift and push your partner's arms forward (**4**).

With your hands on your partner's arms just below the elbows, lean your weight on them and, at the same time, gently push them forwards, elbows away from shoulders (**5**).

Place one hand on the front hip and the other on the back hip. Help your partner to rotate by slowly pushing the front hip and pulling the back hip. Make sure the back heel does not lift off the floor by placing your toes on it (**6**).

Place one hand on the ankle and the other on the top hip bone. Gently and slowly lean your weight on the hip and at the same time lift it upwards towards the wall (**7**).

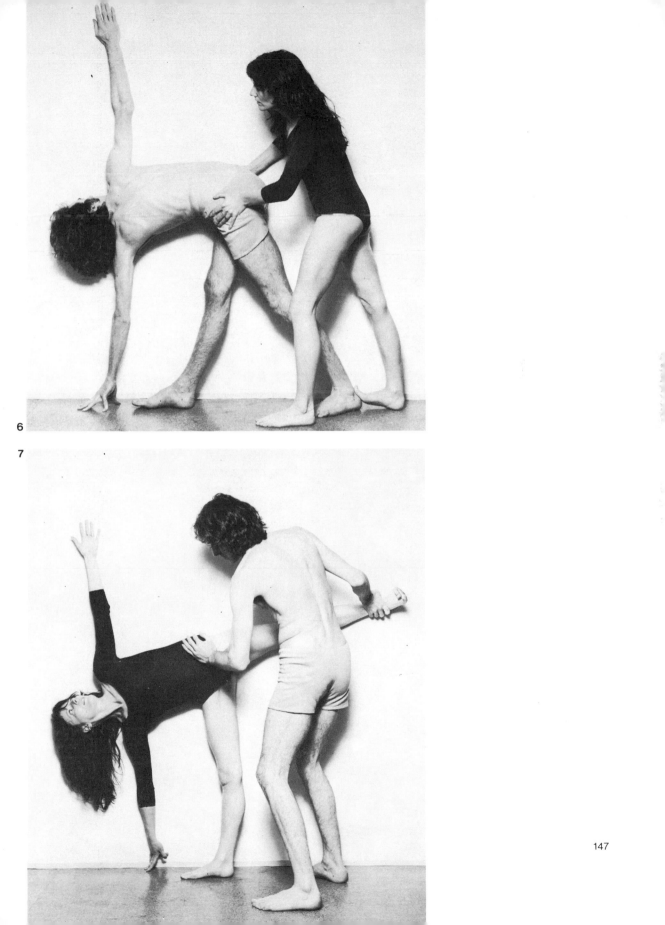

6

7

147

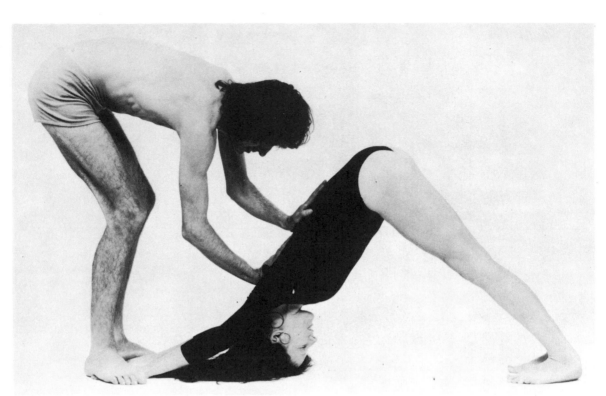

**8**

Place the arches of your feet gently on the fingers and the palms of your hands on the back. Slowly lean your weight without pushing until your partner indicates that it is enough. This position, when cultivated, brings shape to your legs (**8**).

When someone has been practising the tailor position for a long time, you may promote their movement further by using the weight of your legs – or the weight of your entire body (**9a,b**).

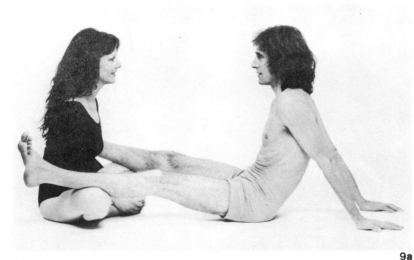

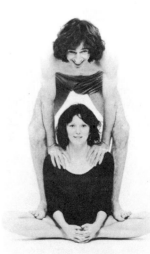

**9a**      **9b**

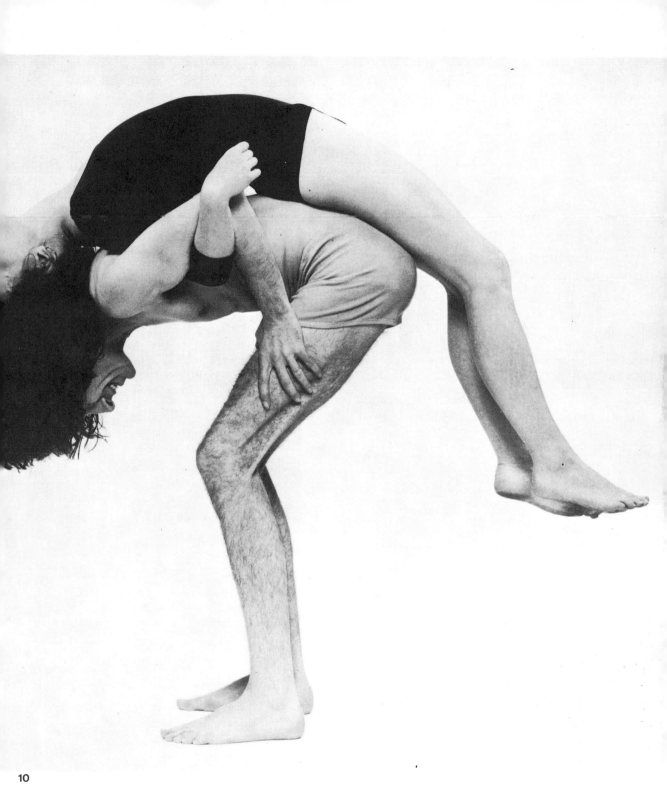

**10**

If your partner's spine is reasonably flexible, this is a very good way to stretch the entire body. Keep your knees bent so as to support the weight without strain (**10**).

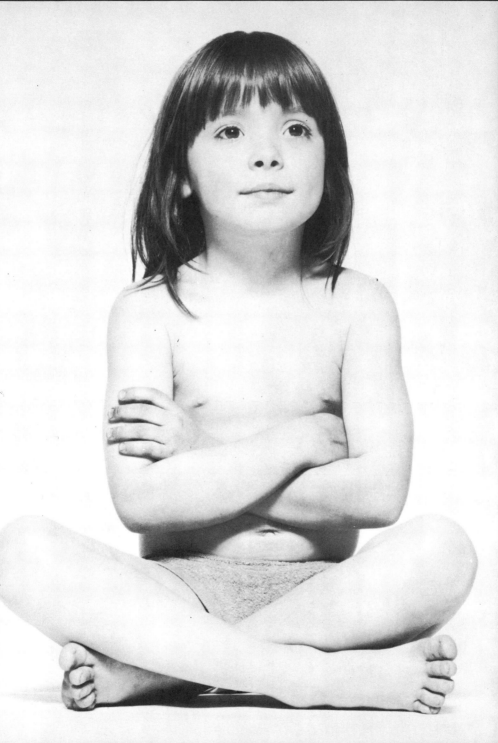

1  Easy sitting

Children love to use their bodies and delight in balancing upside down, cartwheeling and imitating movements, especially those relating to animals. They need very few instructions and should just play and have fun, balancing, moving and imitating the positions as best they can.

Children who are beginning to become stiff usually take a surprisingly short time to regain their suppleness if they play at these positions often enough.

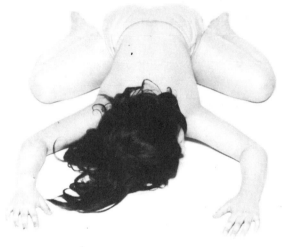

**2 Frog**

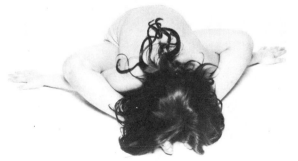

**3 Variation of frog**

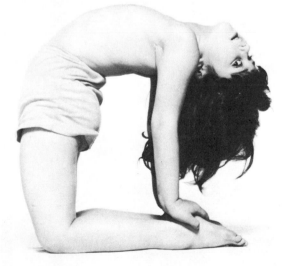

**4 Camel**

**5 Tortoise**

151

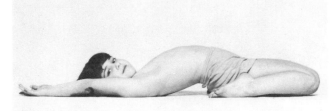

**6 Fish**

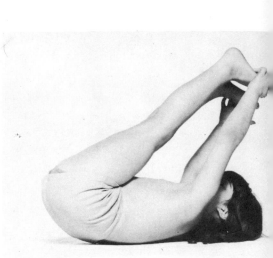

**9 Sloth**

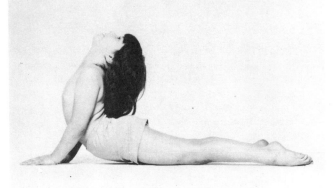

**7 Cobra**

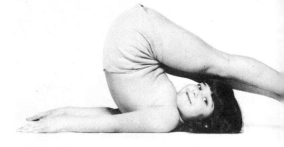

**10 Plough**

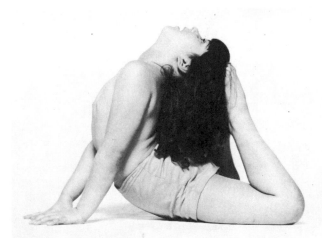

**8 Seal**

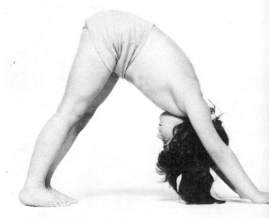

**11 Dog**

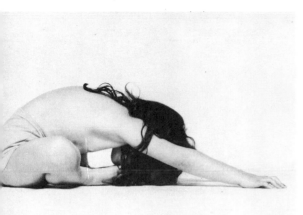

**Butterfly**

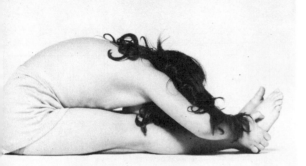

**Jack-knife**

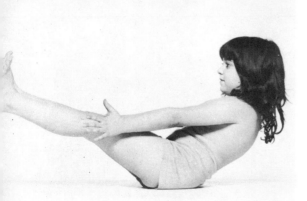

**Boat**

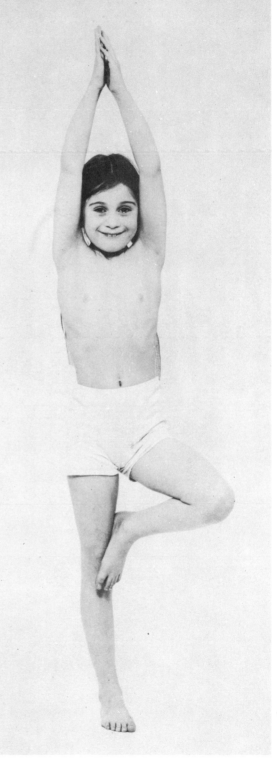

**15 Tree**

153

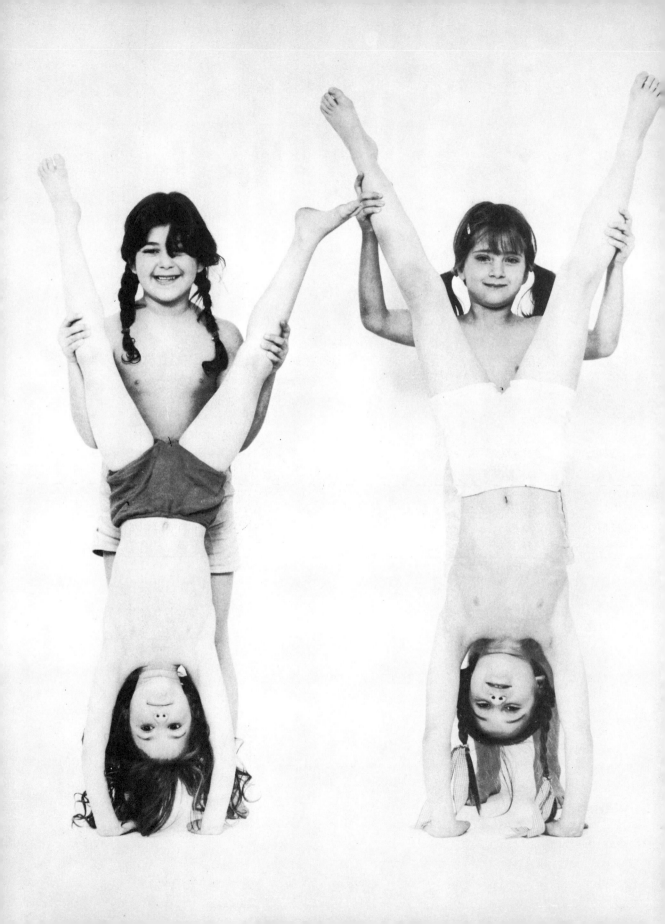

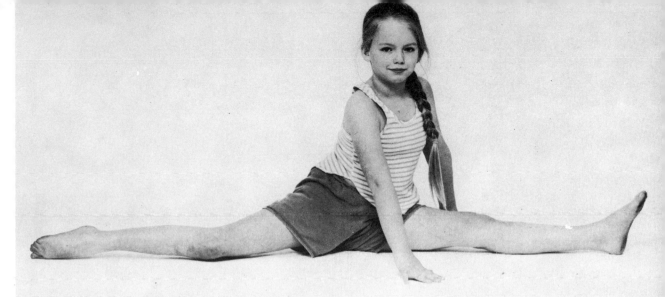

**17 Splits**

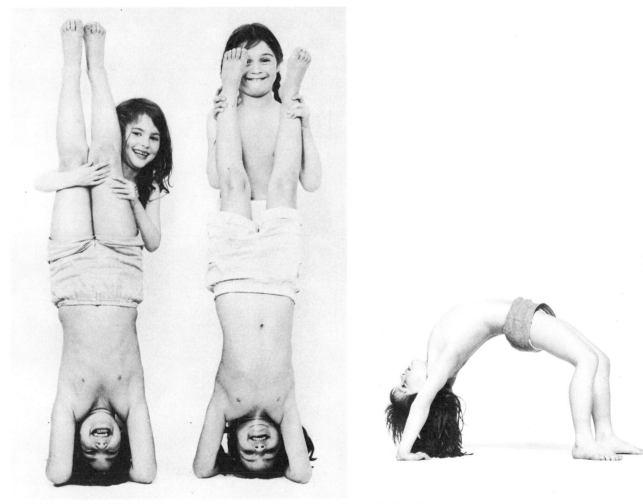

**18 Elbowstand**

**19 Crab**

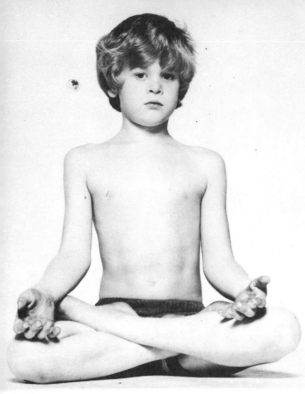

**20 Lotus**

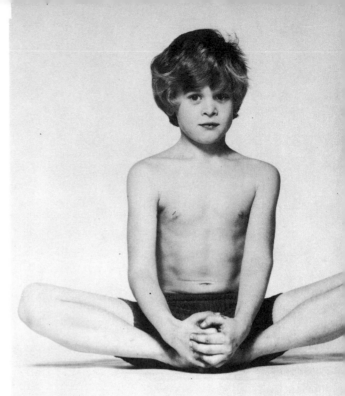

**21 Tailor**

**22 Forward lotus**
**23 Backward lotus**

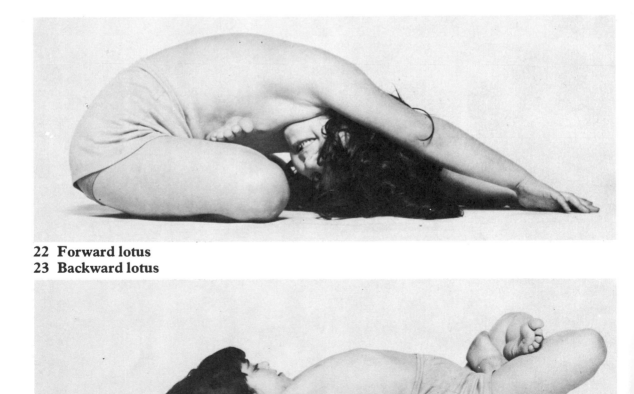

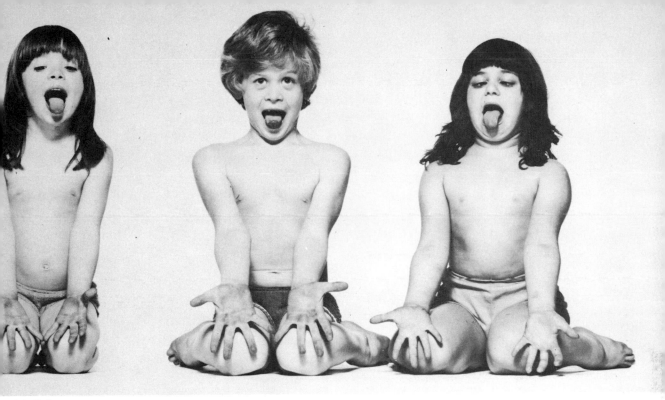

24 Lion
25 Rabbit

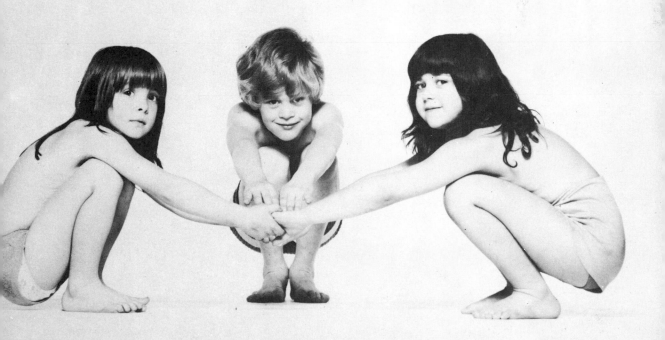

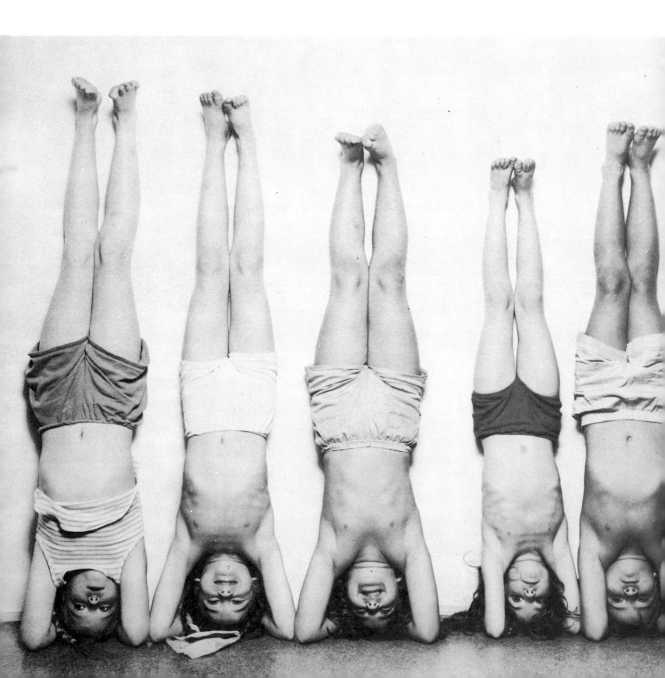

# 18 Movements for pregnant women

## *Preparing to be a mother*

Knowledge of how your reproductive organs work is part of the preparation for giving birth to your child. You should know their position and function, both when you are pregnant and when you are not, and the way they behave during the various stages of labour. Usually during pregnancy you will be under the care of a doctor or an ante-natal clinic and they will give you this information. They will also offer suggestions about the care of your health and diet.

But childbirth is in part a dynamic physical activity and must be prepared for in that context. Therefore, besides all the advice you get from your doctor or clinic we suggest these preparations:

1 Self-massage, especially on the pelvic area of your abdomen and your breasts. Also massage your face, because that relaxes your whole body. Apart from the direct benefit self-massage is also a way of getting to know your body. (See Chapter 4.)

2 Care of your feet. Especially in the later months of pregnancy your feet will have to carry a greater strain, and foot comfort is essential for a happy pregnancy. Carry yourself as erect as possible and stand or walk with your feet parallel to each other. (See Chapter 12 for ways of making your feet flexible.)

3 Undertake a programme of easy, non-strenuous movements. Your body thrives on an intelligent exercise of its possibilities. Joints become stiff with inactivity, supple with proper use, and painful with misuse. Muscles become short and tight with disuse and sleek and beautiful with proper activity.

Movements during pregnancy should include such usual activities as walking, swimming, gardening, and also specific positions to strengthen, relax and prepare the particular muscles that will be used in the actual birth. (Ideally, of course, in preparation for childbirth every muscle, ligament and joint in your body should be supple.)

It is beneficial to make your pelvic joints supple and to tone up and relax the muscles of your pelvic floor in readiness for giving birth. The prescribed movements will help you to obtain the maximum capacity for your pelvis, thereby giving the baby plenty of room.

A flexible spine prevents backache caused by the strain on the muscles of your back during the later months of pregnancy, when your pelvis holds the increasing weight of the baby. Also the force which the contracting uterus exerts in lengthening the spinal ligaments and muscles during labour produces considerable strain unless care has been taken to maintain their normal flexibility.

Below your pubic bones is your sub-pubic arch and it is from under this arch that the baby's head comes through at birth. Therefore, it is advisable to practise movements which will widen this arch to its maximum to make the front wall of the birth canal as short as possible. The squatting postures have a strong widening effect.

The squatting position is our instinctive toilet posture. It also stretches naturally the genital areas that will be stretched in childbirth and increases the flow of blood to these parts. (Eskimos and many other races give birth in this position.) Use this position whenever possible when going to the toilet; it places far less strain on your inner organs.

Relaxation of the floor of your pelvis and widening of its structures are aided by movements in which your knees are parted and your pelvic floor widened sideways – movements in which the pelvis is at its widest. A tight and rigid pelvic floor delays the arrival of the baby.

All the movements must be carried out slowly, smoothly and rhythmically. Begin with a small range and gradually increase as you become proficient. To get the full value it is essential that you practise some of them each day throughout pregnancy. Your clothing should be loose and you should have a blanket on the floor to sit or lie on.

## Pre-natal positions and movements

### Movements 1 and 2: Squatting

Standing with feet slightly apart, grasp a support. Rise on tiptoe and lower your body into the squatting position: your knees widely parted, your head and back erect. Now rock back on to your heels (**1,2**). The parting of your knees relaxes the adductors on your inner thighs and increases the width of your sub-pubic arch and your pelvic floor outlet. Go into the squat position ten times at first and build up to many more, on other occasions stay in the position for a few minutes.

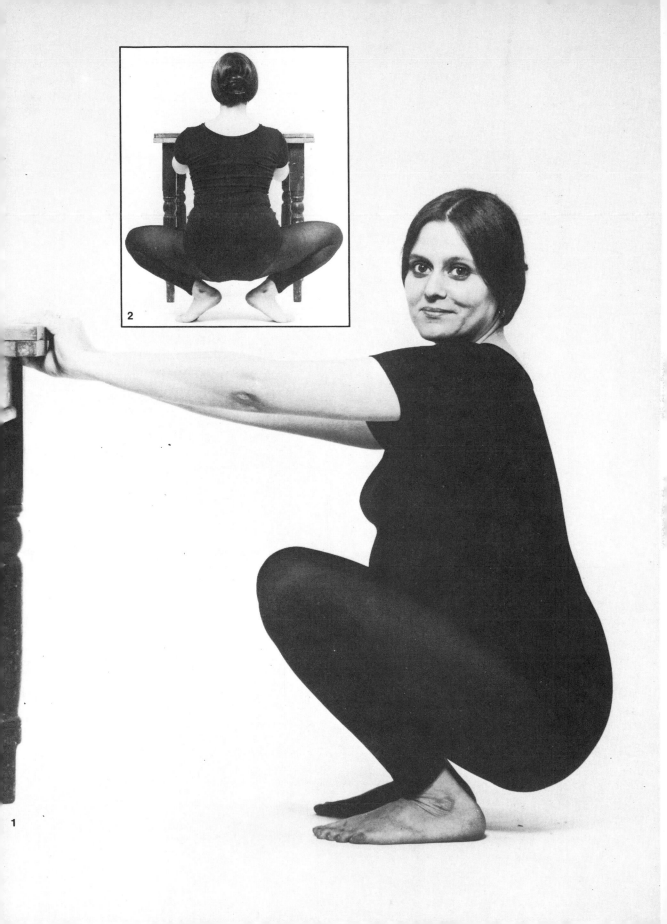

1

2

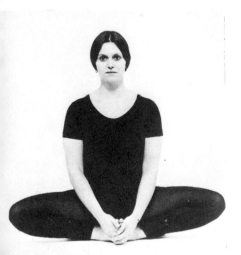

### Movement 3: The tailor position

Sit with knees bent out, the soles of your feet together and your hands grasping your ankles. A cushion may be used to straighten your back. Timing is essential for the cultivation of this movement, which widens, lengthens, stretches and tones your pelvic floor and relaxes your inner thighs.

### Movement 4

Sit on your heels. Now, taking your feet to the sides, sit on the floor. If this is difficult, try sitting on a cushion. Make sure your toes turn slightly inwards and your heels outwards.

### Movement 5

Now in this position spread your knees as wide as possible. Each day spend a minute or two in these two positions until you can eventually sit in each of them for 5 minutes with ease and comfort.

3

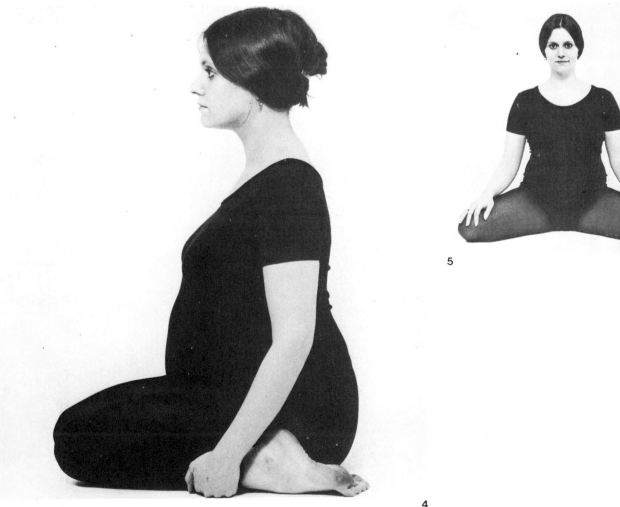

5

4

## Movement 6

Sitting on your heels, extend your arms out to your sides, with palms facing downwards. Now turn your palms upwards and backwards so that both arms rotate as far as they can. Hold for 15 seconds and rest. Repeat this as many times a day as you wish.

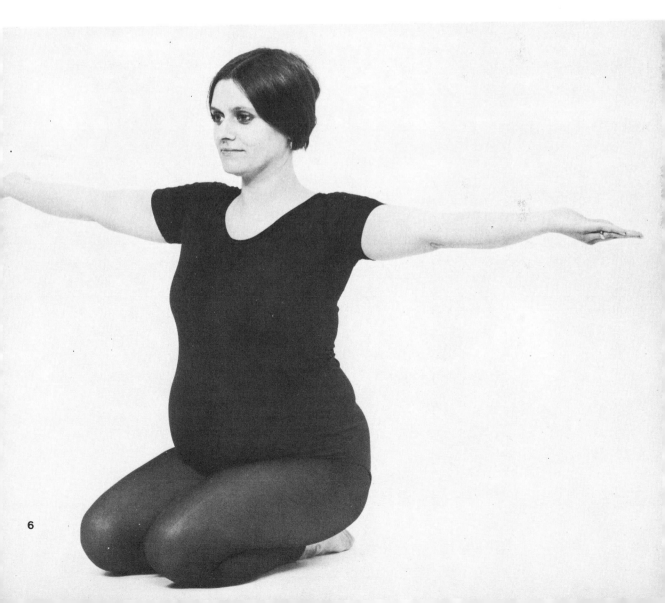

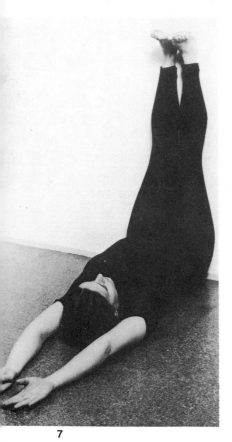

## Movement 7

Lie on your back with your buttocks against the wall and your legs on the wall. Either keep your knees straight or bend your knees as much as possible, with your feet on the wall. Take your arms overhead, hands extended, keeping your elbows straight and firm. Lie in this position for a minute at first and build up to 5 minutes.

By making sure your lower back remains in contact with the floor, your back is supported. If your pectorals are tight your arms will not make complete contact with the floor. When they do, your pectorals are sufficiently long and relaxed.

## Movement 8

Lie on your back with your buttocks against the wall and your legs straight on the wall. Slowly spread your legs apart as far as they will go comfortably. Keep your knees extended but not tight and do not point your toes.

This simple movement lengthens your inner thigh muscles and widens your sub-pubic arch and pelvic floor outlet. Your back is supported and safe, but since these muscles are very large and strong use caution in how long you lengthen them. If it is not too demanding, you can also extend your arms overhead.

This is a very good position for massaging and exploring your groin and the bones of your pelvis, especially the sub-pubic arch.

7

8

## Movement 9: The pelvic tilt

Lie on your back on the floor comfortably, with knees flexed and feet on the ground. First contract your abdominal muscles as hard as possible. Then rest. Contract your buttock muscles. Rest. Now contract both your abdominal and buttock muscles, making a pelvic tilt with flexion of your lower back, the small of your back pressing against the floor.

When you can do this, the contractions should be held as long as possible. At first you may manage only 10 seconds or so, but you should build up to at least 20 seconds to complete the exercise. To start with you may not find it possible to breathe normally when contracting the muscles to the maximum, but as you become accustomed to the movement your breathing will return to normal.

Once you have mastered this basic movement, you may carry it out standing, sitting, lying and even when you are walking. This means it can be done regularly and repeatedly.

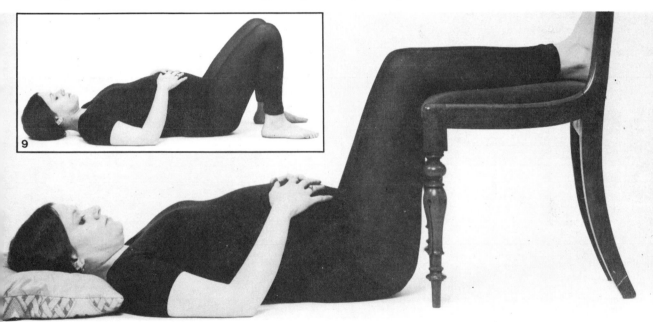

## Movement 10

Lie down with a pillow under your head and your feet on a chair. This is a very good resting position. Now, with eyes open or closed, go through your entire body, trying to feel it proprioceptively.

That is, not thinking about how you feel — not whether you are happy or depressed or bored – but the actual sense of feeling in various parts of your body. Feel from within all the parts of your body. Start with your feet and work upwards to your head, face and finally eyes. The secret of successful resting is self-awareness.

# 19 Backache

What kind of exercise to use in the treatment of backache has always been a controversial question.

Probably the most widely known and practised are 'back extension' exercises, perhaps because it is thought that the spinal extensors exert the most effect in maintaining spinal posture. Most of these movements emphasize using the extensor muscles of the spine to resist gravity. They are done lying on the floor on your back and front. They directly strengthen the muscles of your back – on much the same principle as in weight-lifting.

Less well known, but also widely used, are 'active flexion' exercises, including toe-touching. But these have been criticized as producing permanently unstable and irritable joints.

Others prefer abdominal strengthening exercises such as straight-leg raising, lying on your back. Other techniques aim to raise intra-abdominal pressure.

Most of these techniques miss very important points.

Firstly, they deal directly with the muscles of the spine, overlooking the fact that the lumbar joints do not act alone but in close relationship with the joints of the hip. If the hip joints are stiff and inflexible the strain and load of trunk movement usually fall on the lumbar vertebrae. The hip joints, being larger and stronger, do not weaken or collapse before the lumbar joints. Therefore, to lessen the strain on the lumbar joints you have to create better movement and flexibility of the hip joints and the muscle groups which operate them.

The same applies to the upper back in relation to the shoulders. Free the shoulder muscles and joints, and only then work directly on the upper back. To work on the muscles of the spine before those of the hips and shoulders is dangerous.

Another point is overlooked: strengthening muscles to resist weight may prevent collapse of those muscles under strain, but will never release the prolonged contraction and thus tension of those muscles. The theory of these methods is that your back is collapsing under strain, so make it strong enough to resist that collapse. This may stop further deterioration, but it certainly does not promote flexibility and relaxation of the muscles.

If you have constant lower back pain, examine and give special attention to the following: your general posture; the angle of your lumbar curve and whether this is exaggerated;

the tone and power of your abdominal and hip flexor muscles; the stiffness of your hip joints and of your lumbar spine when actively moving them. Remember that taken as a whole your lumbar vertebrae should function as a 'universal joint'.

To treat backache we must first begin with exercises for the hips and shoulders—movements assisted by the force of gravity, without any direct strain on the back itself. Only after these joints have become reasonably supple can you proceed to work directly on the spine. And then you do this always aided by the force of gravity in every movement.

The movements are very simple, non-strenuous exercises which should be carried out several times a day on your own. Frequent repetition of a movement is far better than a lengthy exercise period. Throughout the day also try to keep your knees slightly flexed, rather than rigid, and your body straight and easy, especially when lifting, standing or walking.

Sudden or severe attacks of backache may call for some preparatory action before the exercises can begin.

Many people have tender spots on their bodies ('trigger spots'), especially in the neck, shoulders, upper and lower back and hip muscles, which are caused by strain or spasm. These painful spots have to be massaged gently away with the help of heat. Tenderness of the skin—fibrositis—may respond to gentle pinching massage over a long period.

If you should suffer an attack of back pain, try a hot pack made up of a towel dipped in hot water, wrung out completely and then wrapped in a dry towel. Lie down on a firm surface and cover the painful muscles with the hot pack. The sudden heat seems to shock the muscles and helps to relieve the pain. Ice packs are also helpful. While it is important to rest whenever possible, gentle limbering up should be continued to avoid unnecessary stiffening of the afflicted area.

Once the various pains have gone, the therapeutic movements can then be practised.

In all the following, simple, non-strenuous movements in muscle relaxing, assistance is the name of the game. You are simply assisting natural movements to their anatomical limit.

## The pelvic tilt

The cause of much lower back pain is an exaggerated hollow in the lumbar spine. This may be the result of bad habits in bending or of stiff hip joints. For example, if you bend down to pick up something from the floor, if your joints are in good condition you will bend primarily at the hip joints and only secondly at the lumbar joints. But if your joints are immobile, the hip joints will lock and remain unyielding while the lumbar joints are used in a way for which they were not designed.

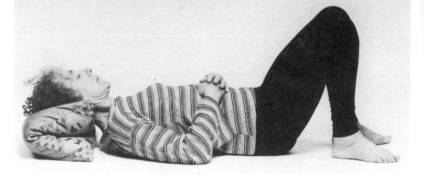

The only lasting way to bring ease to this area is to exercise the hip joints. But the pelvic tilt exercise or lumbar flexion technique – well known in the traditions of Hatha Yoga and Zen sitting – will help if used in conjunction with exercises to free the hip joints.

Lie on your back on the floor comfortably, with knees flexed and feet on the ground. First, contract your abdominal muscles as hard as possible. Then relax. Contract your buttock muscles. Relax. Now contract both your abdominal and buttock muscles, making a pelvic tilt with flexion of your lumbar spine, so that the small of your back presses against the floor.

When you can do this, the contractions should be held as long as possible. At first, you may manage only 10 seconds or so, but you should build up to at least 20 seconds to complete the exercise. Increase both the duration of the contraction and the number of times it is carried out. To start with you may not find it possible to breathe normally when contracting the muscles to the maximum, but as you become accustomed to the movement your breathing will return to normal.

When the movement is easy, try it with arms extended over your head.

One of the greatest advantages of this lumbar flexion movement or pelvic tilt is its simplicity. You only have to master the basic movement and you can carry it out standing, sitting, lying, even while you are walking, and so on. This means that it can be done regularly and repeatedly.

With much practice this movement eventually realigns the lumbar vertebrae and establishes their lost relationship with the hip joints. Probably the most likely reason why this movement is so helpful is that it involves only a minimum of movement in the spinal structures, which are therefore not strained.

It must be pointed out that this movement is not a panacea for all forms of lower back pain. It is only an assisting adjunct to other movements and positions. Its prime importance is for people with exaggerated lower backs and lax abdominal muscles.

The following movements may safely be practised by the elderly and the very stiff as well as back pain sufferers.

# Movements for your shoulders and neck

Tension headache, stiff neck, tense shoulders and upper back pain are all intimately connected. The cultivation of a few simple movements will help to ease these pains.

The principal muscles holding your head upright are those at the back and sides of your neck. You can feel them contracting if you place the palm of your hand on the back of your head and then, moving your head backwards and chin upwards, resist the movement with your other hand. These muscles are constantly at work in the upright position. It is no wonder that they are so often stiff and short. If you lower your head they lengthen – if you lift your head they shorten. For some reason many people hold their chins slightly upwards, so tilting their heads backwards. This not only strains the neck muscles but places the joints in a very dangerous situation. A slight jolt or sudden turn or twist in this unstable position results in a stiff neck or painful shoulders or a tension headache.

## Movement 1
Take a stool with a cushion on it. Now lie down with your head a foot or so away from it. Bend your knees and with your hands as support lift your trunk off the ground. Then slowly straighten your legs until they rest on the stool.

At first hold this position for about half a minute. With practice you should gradually be able to remain in it with ease for 5 minutes. In this position you use the weight and leverage of your trunk and legs to lengthen, stretch and relax the overworked shoulder and neck muscles.

When the position has become easy try taking your hands overhead. Then add another variation by extending your arms backwards with hands interlocked. This lengthens your shoulder and chest muscles. The occipital muscle groups at the back of your head are also relaxed and, because they work in conjunction with your eye muscles, the eyes in time become less tense.

1

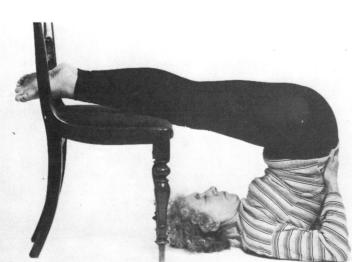

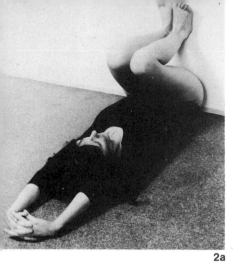

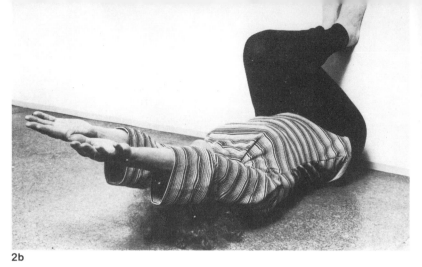

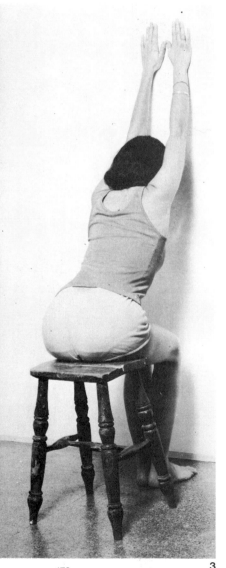

2a    2b

### Movement 2

Lie on your back with your legs on a wall, forming an L with your trunk and legs. Now bend your knees as much as possible, with your feet on the wall. Take your arms overhead, keeping your elbows straight and firm. Ask someone to stand behind you to hold your arms to prevent them from coming forward. Resist for a few seconds and feel which muscles of your chest and shoulders contract. Relax and then extend your arms overhead. The muscle groups that you felt contracting are now being stretched and relaxed. Lie in this position for a minute and build up to 5 minutes (**2a**).

In this position your back is supported. Make sure your lumbar vertebrae or lower back remains in contact with the floor. If your pectoral muscles are tight your arms will not make complete contact with the floor (**2b**). When they do, your pectorals are sufficiently long and relaxed.

### Movement 3

This position relaxes and lengthens the same muscles as the last movement. Place a chair facing a wall, a few feet away from it. Sit on the edge of the chair with your feet firmly on the ground. Now extend your arms overhead and lean against the wall. Or sit on your feet with knees apart and lean on the wall.

Here you use the weight of your body against the wall to lengthen your front chest and shoulder muscle groups. Don't force, rather let go and relax. Start at a minute and build up to 5. For variety, try different positions of your head, hanging forward or level and straight.

### Movement 4

Place a mat or thick folded blanket on a solid table. Lie on your back so that just your head falls back with the pull of gravity. Your knees should be flexed with your feet on the wall, to ensure that your lower back lies firmly on the table. Let your arms rest by your sides. Keep your lower jaw closed against your upper jaw. Do not open your mouth or you will not get the proper throat stretch.

Stay in this position for about half a minute and very slowly in stages build up your time to 5 minutes.

When coming out of this position move very slowly and turn on to your side.

### Movement 5

Starting in the same position, jut your head a little further out and take your arms overhead with hands interlocked. Master this stage and then jut your head still further over the edge of the table, a little at a time. Stay in each stage as long as is comfortable until you build up to 5 minutes.

All the front muscles of the top half of your body are being lengthened and relaxed with assistance from gravity, and without resistance, strain or stress on your lower back. Do not be in a rush. The longer you take in each stage the better. This is the only safe way to extend your spine and stretch the front muscle groups of your body.

You will realize how vital this exercise is when you think how much of your day you spend hunched forward and how much of your life you have spent like that. Continually hunched up, your front muscles shorten and lose their ability to lengthen. The only way to bring life to your frontal body muscle groups is passively to lengthen them in order to release their tension and prolonged contraction. It is safe to do this exercise if you proceed with caution and care. Aim only at gradual progress and, once more, always make sure that your lower back does not lift from the table.

4    5

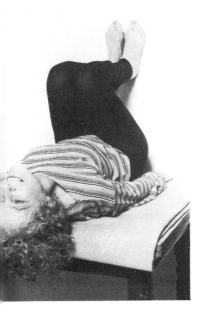

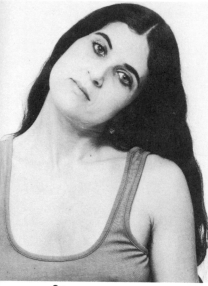

6a

## Movement 6

Sitting, keeping your chin slightly in and at the centre line of your body, gently place your ear as near as possible to your right shoulder (**6a**). This lengthens the trapezius muscle of the opposite side. Then do the same on the left side. To start with, hold your extreme position for 15 seconds and build up to 2 minutes on each side. Then, keeping your chin slightly in, rotate or twist your head first to the left then to the right (**6b**). Hold each side for half a minute and build up to 2 minutes on each side.

## Movement 7

Sit on a chair with feet together. With hips firm, twist or rotate your body as much as possible with the help of your hands, first to the left. Hold for 10 seconds. Relax and then rotate your body to the right. Hold for 10 seconds. Build up to a minute on each side in the extreme position. These movements stem from your upper chest vertebrae.

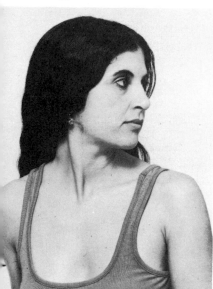

6b

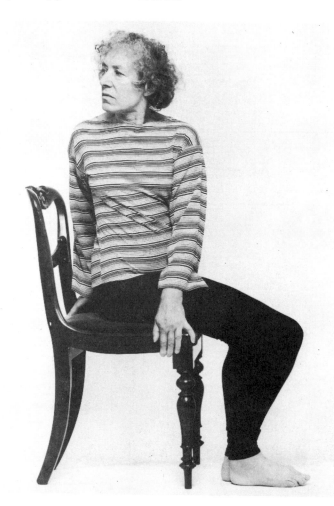

7

# *Movements for your hips and lower back*

Now for the simplest hip movements that lengthen and relax the muscles operating on your hip joints.

### Movement 1

Lie on your back, buttocks against a wall and your legs together up the wall, forming an L. Keep your hands at your sides, and if your chin protrudes place a small cushion behind your head to avoid straining your neck. From your L position, flex one knee and with your hands, bring it as close as possible to your chest. Repeat with the other leg.

### Movement 2

Bend your knees, bringing them towards your chest, feet on the wall. Stay in this position as long as you like. It is a safe one. Your back is supported and gravity or the weight of your legs is assisting the movement. When this becomes easy you can use your hands to pull your knees in further. This often helps very quickly in alleviating severe lower back pain.

Remember the emphasis is on aiding the contracting muscles to shorten and the relaxing muscles to lengthen, in any and every movement.

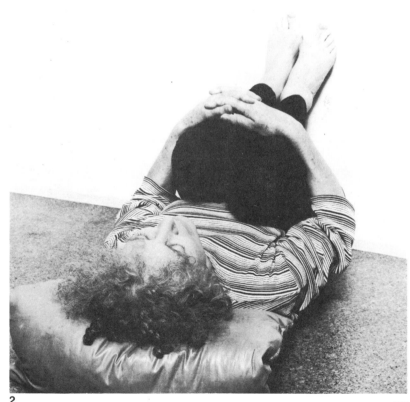

1

2

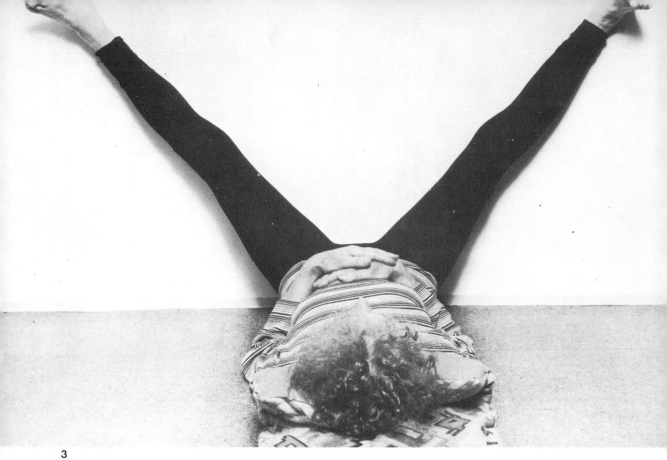

3

## Movement 3

From your L position, slowly spread your legs apart as far as they will go. Keep your knees extended but not tight and do not point your toes.

This simple movement lengthens and stretches your inner thigh muscles, the adductors. Your back is supported and safe, but since the muscles are very large and strong be careful not to stretch them for too long when you begin. Stay in the position only as long as it is comfortable.

## Movement 4

In your L position, take a belt and place it around your right ankle. Now, keeping your knee straight, bring the leg to you, helping it by pulling gently on the belt. Your entire back and neck should be relaxed; if necessary place a cushion behind your head. You don't need a belt if you can interlock your hands behind your knee or hold your foot and gently assist the leg forward. Do the same equally for both legs. This exercise lengthens and relaxes the hamstring group of muscles.

Again, your back is supported and safe, so that the only stretch will be in your hamstrings. When this becomes relatively easy try the next movement.

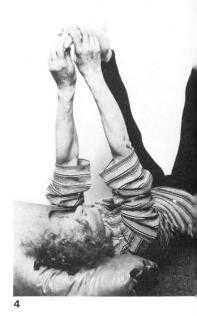

4

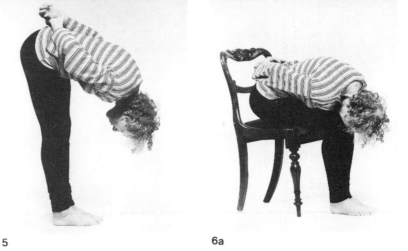

5

6a

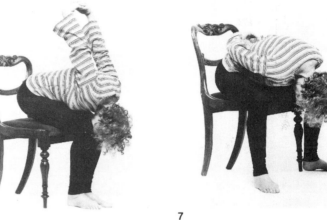

6b

7

## Movement 5
Stand up, clasp your hands behind your back, keeping your back and neck straight. Gradually lower your trunk, bending from your hips, and go down as far as you can until you feel your hamstring muscles stretching. The weight of your trunk assists the action, helping the hip flexors to contract, lengthening the hamstrings. There should be no pain or ache in your lower back. If there is stop at once and go back to Movement Four.

## Movement 6
Sit on a chair, feet together on the floor. Drop your trunk forward as far as you can (**6a**). Stay like that as long as it is comfortable and then straighten up. This can be done many times a day in your office or at home.

Try clasping your hands and extending your arms backwards (**6b**). Hold for 15 seconds and repeat a few times.

## Movement 7
Try it with feet apart. Drop your neck, shoulders, arms, then bend down towards your knees as far as you can.

Another variation is to bend down to the left, straighten up and do the same on the right.

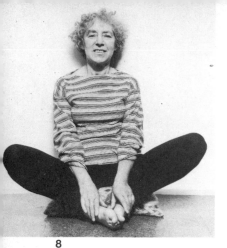

8

### Movement 8

Sit with your back against a wall and your legs straight in front of you. Again it is an L position, but the reverse of the previous L. Now bend your knees and bring your feet in as close as possible to your body, holding them together with your hands.

The back is supported by the wall and the weight of flexed knees stretches and relaxes your thigh muscles. Stay in this position as long as you find comfortable. Build up your time gradually from, say, 30 seconds to 5 minutes. If this is very difficult start with a cushion under your seat. This helps straighten your back.

### Movement 9

Sitting between your legs is an important movement as it lengthens some of the articular muscles of your hip by rotating your thighs inwards (**9a**). If you find this difficult, begin by sitting on your feet (**9b**). Together this movement and the previous one (the tailor position, which rotates your thighs outwards) lengthen and relax all the articular muscles of your hips.

### Movement 10

Find something that can support your full body-weight. Hold on to it and with feet apart gradually go into a squatting position. Hold for 10 seconds and then slowly straighten up. Gradually build up the time you can do this with ease. Then bring your feet closer together until you can do the movement with feet together.

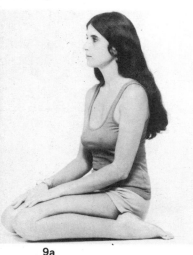

9a

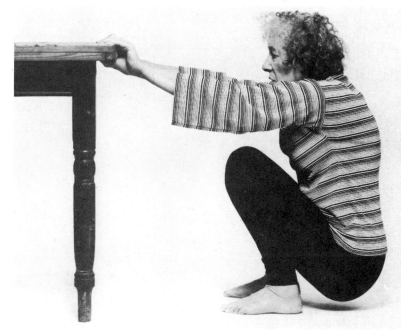

9b

10

## Sleeping positions

People who suffer from backache are often awakened by pain during the night and are usually very stiff in the morning. The position in which they have been sleeping is often to blame. Change to a position that results in flexion rather than extension of your lower back. A firm mattress should be used to give full support to your trunk so that it can relax.

If you sleep face down, of course, your lower back curve is considerably increased, especially if you sleep on a very stiff mattress. Change to an alternative posture, but if you find it difficult to sleep in any other position place a small pillow under one hip so that your lumber spine is not completely extended.

If you sleep on your side with one knee bent, place a small cushion under your knee so that it does not fall into a position that puts an unnecessary strain on your back.

If you prefer to lie flat on your back it is advisable to tilt your head with pillows forming a wedge position so that your shoulders are supported. Your back then automatically assumes a flexed position.

If you lie flat on your back your lumbar spine is usually extended in an exaggerated way. Place a long, narrow cushion under your knees to help to flex your lumbar spine.

If you wake up with lower back pain during the night or in the morning on rising, curl up with knees on your chest and your head flexed forward. This stretches the lumbar spine.

If your back is very stiff, heat, either from a hot-water bottle or electric blanket, can help it. It is especially useful before getting up in the morning.

If you wake up with a stiff neck or tense, stiff shoulders, you have probably slept in a position in which your chin is lifted and your shoulders rounded. If you sleep on your side and on your front, try to keep your head and chin slightly in. If you sleep on your back prop up your head slightly with a small cushion.

# 20 Exercises in the office

The following is a selection of simple exercises that can be done in the office.

## Movement 1: Squatting
Hold on to a solid table or desk and go into a squatting position. Make sure your back is straight and your heels are on the floor. Repeat ten times and build up to many more.

## Movement 2: To lengthen and relax your hamstring muscles
Standing with your feet about a foot apart, bend forward with your hands joined on your buttocks. Hold your left wrist with your right hand or vice versa. Lever your pelvis and trunk forward. Do not bend your back or neck too much; just allow your body to hang forward without using any effort. The weight of your trunk as a lever lengthens the back of your thighs, especially behind your knees. Begin with half a minute at a time, and build up to 5 or 10 minutes.

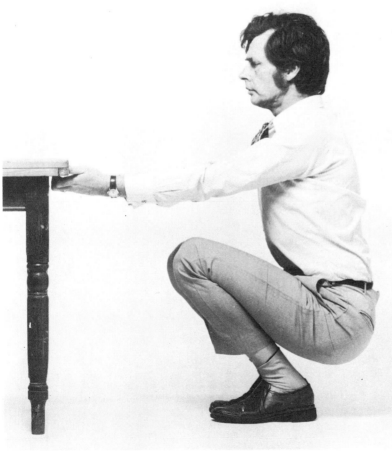

1

## Movement 3

Sit on a chair, feet together on the floor. Take your hands behind your back, one hand gripping the wrist of the other. Drop your trunk forward as far as you can. Stay like this for as long as is comfortable, building up to 5 minutes.

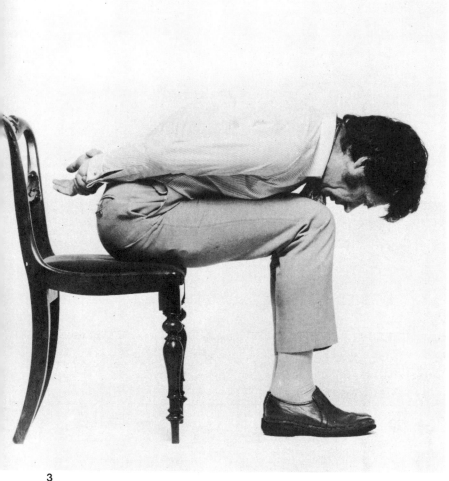

3

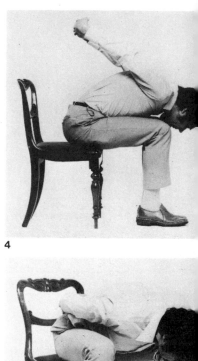

4

5

## Movement 4: Bending your arms backwards

Sitting on a chair, bend forward with arms going backwards as far as possible and hands interlocked. Ask someone to assist the movement, if possible – just a gentle pull. Hold for about 20 seconds at a time.

## Movement 5

Try it with your feet apart. Take your hips and trunk downwards towards the floor.

Another variation is to bend down on the left thigh, hold for 30 seconds, straighten up and do the same on the right.

180

## Movement 6: To rotate your arms

Sitting comfortably on a chair, extend your arms out to your sides, with palms facing downwards. Now bring your palms upwards and backwards so that both arms rotate as far as they can. Hold for 20 seconds and release. Repeat this as many times a day as you wish.

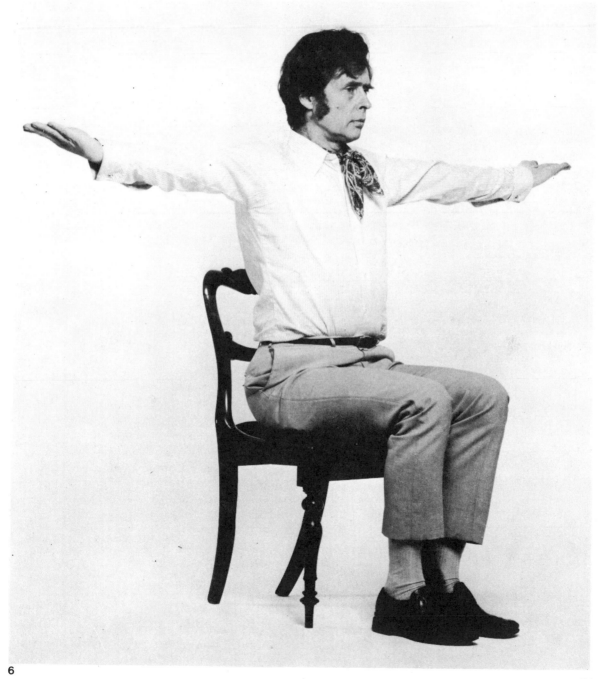

6

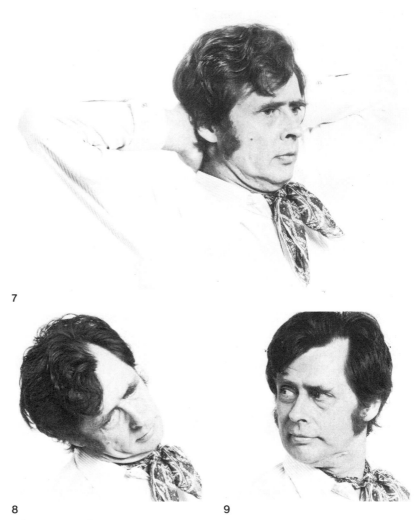

7

8                                          9

**Movement 7**
Sitting or standing interlock your hands behind your head and
take your elbows as far back as possible.

**Movement 8: To bend your neck sideways**
Sitting or standing, keep your chin slightly in and at the centre
line of your body. Now gently place your ear as near as possible
to your right shoulder. Do not raise your shoulder. Now do the
same on the left.

    This movement lengthens and relaxes the trapezius
muscles. It can be done many times a day.

**Movement 9: To rotate your head**
Centre your head with your chin slightly in and rotate your
head to the left, as if you were trying to look behind you. Hold
for a few seconds, gently rotating as much as possible. Repeat
on the left side. This, too, can be done many times every day.

**Movement 10**

Sitting or standing, take one hand overhead, bending your arm backwards to meet the other arm going down and backwards, as in the photograph. Repeat with hands reversed. Don't be discouraged if your hands do not meet at first, with practice they eventually will.

**Movement 11**

Take both hands behind your back so that your palms face each other as in the photograph. Take your elbows backwards and keep your trunk straight. Hold as long as it is comfortable.

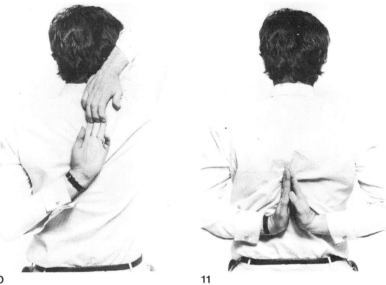

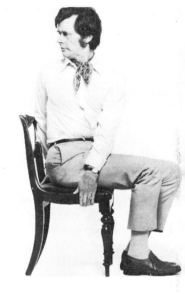

10                            11                            12

**Movement 12**

Sit on a chair. With hips firm, twist or rotate your body as much as possible with the help of your hands holding the sides of the chair, as in the photograph. First to the left. Hold for 15 seconds. Rest and then rotate your body to the right. Build up to one minute on each side.

**Movement 13: To lengthen and relax your breast muscles**

Sit on the edge of a chair with feet apart a few feet away from a wall. Extend your arms on to the wall as in the photograph. Your elbows should be straight and your hands about shoulder width apart. Don't force, rather let go and relax. Start at a minute and build up to 5 minutes.

Here you use the weight of your body against the wall to lengthen your front shoulder muscles.

Finally, with your eyes open or closed, massage your forehead, temples, eyes, cheekbones, the bridge of your nose, your lower jaw, and so on (see Chapter 4).

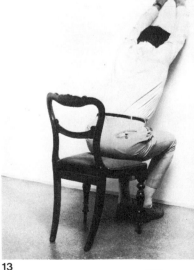

13

# 21 How people benefit

As this book has emphasized throughout, there is no instant way of restoring a misused body to its full potential. The movements are easy to follow and they are not strenuous, but there will be occasions when bringing muscles back into use will be painful for a time – the beneficial pain explained in Chapter 3. But if the movements are mastered gradually so that one stage can be carried out comfortably before passing on to the next, and if the movements are done regularly, there is no doubt of the ultimate benefit.

Readers may find helpful and reassuring the following experiences of a few of my students, especially with regard to the difficulties they encountered and their progress in overcoming them.

When I first met my wife she had been doing yoga for five years. She told me that not having tried it myself I couldn't possibly cling to my impression that it was something mysteriously practised by priests, gurus or circus performers. She showed me a few movements, but I was quite embarrassed at the difficulty my body had in trying to make them, and I was not prepared to spend the time or effort necessary for improvement.

I was thirty years old and had been a hairdresser since the age of seventeen. This involved long hours of standing and bending over people's hair. The inevitable happened – severe pain in my lower back. At first I tried to ignore it, but as the pain increased, I sought the help of a doctor and a chiropractor and started daily swimming. My health improved enormously, but at the end of a year I was still suffering from my back pain.

As a last resort I decided to give this yoga another try. I joined Arthur's class and quickly learned to focus attention on my body itself and not on yoga as a system.

The fact that other people could make beautifully natural movements and I couldn't amazed me. After a while, I overcame my shyness about being stiff and started to become excited by my new discovery. As I got more into every lesson it would leave me feeling full of well-being. I was now practising daily by myself. I still got the occasional twinge from my back but less severely and not so often.

After a few months I really began to feel my body loosen up and start coming to life. My back pain disappeared completely. What had started as a curative experiment to relieve pain was now becoming a way of life. For the first time since a child I was beginning to understand what a healthy body really meant. I stopped smoking, the newfound feeling of relaxation took the place of nicotine.

This ease and comfort in my body made me more alert and aware of things going on around me, a new level of consciousness through the body. My self-confidence improved, and my relationships with other people. So the essence is this, in eighteen months through giving my body the proper attention it deserves my whole feeling towards life has changed, my confidence, awareness, the senses all are infinitely better and improving all the time.

**John Stirk, hairdresser**

When I began doing yoga, I was very floppy. I could fall into a backbend, but by no means could I slowly lower myself back, and it was only with terrible effort that I could pull myself away from the floor and stand up again. It seemed I could only let go, so for me, learning yoga meant getting a hold of myself.

But then I got almost as stuck in holding on as I had been in my floppiness. I often went completely rigid in my poses, and exhausted myself. I knew I shouldn't, and I started wondering why I was putting myself through so much pain. Fortunately, I was given the very good advice not to try so hard, and as a result, there is much less pain these days and I am rarely exhausted.

Instead, I feel I have more energy. My body has taken on shape and direction; I move more in the poses and feel more confident in all my movements, not just in yoga. I enjoy my body more, and think about it less. The less effort I make, the more I can move, and the more I move, the less effort it takes; the less I want, the more I seem to get. It's a good feeling.

**Barbara Stein**

Yoga for me is a process of self-discovery, both exciting and painful. In the past I've given little thought to my body except when ill. Through yoga I'm beginning to realize the way in which my body is capable of moving and working. It has helped to focus my attention on the stiffness and tension I carry around with me. Yet the yoga also provides a way of relieving this pain and tightness. I've found that I'm now moving and working in a different way. It's a wonderful sensation to walk with a new sense of balance.

Having played a musical instrument for fifteen years, I

assumed my hands would be flexible. Through yoga and massage I've found that they aren't. As their flexibility improves so does my awareness of my hands and music also grow. The warmth that massage has brought to my feet is truly amazing. My feet, which I have taken for granted for so long, are now more sensitive, and as a result, I'm more conscious of the contact between my feet and the ground.

After a yoga session my body feels warm, relaxed and cleansed.

**Karl Schurr, musician**

Throughout my childhood, I was told to be careful every time I moved. Consequently, before I began to do yoga, I was afraid to move. After eighteen months, doing a few exercises every day, I have gradually moved into my body and find it to be a very comfortable and ingeniously designed abode. I am happier, lighter and more attractive. My sexual life has improved immensely. I have more friends and enjoy living and moving. I like myself more – the more I possess my body.

**Janet Hope, ante-natal teacher**

I first started to practise yoga some five years ago. I realized from the first lesson how tense I was and how little I knew myself. I had thought that I was always fairly relaxed, and I wondered whether my wife or friends could see the tension that I then realized I'd been trying to ignore. For eighteen months or so I continued to practise yoga spasmodically. I went to three different teachers before I met Arthur Balaskas. He has been my friend and teacher for some three years now and over that period of time I feel that my awareness of my physical and mental self has changed considerably. Through his help I have regained my sense of self that was lost so long ago I'd forgotten I'd ever had it.

**Peter Walker, company director**

When I came to London in September 1972 to train as a psychotherapist, I was recommended to try Hatha Yoga. In the classes I was one of the people who were 'tight all over'. I could not touch my toes, I could not sit cross-legged, I was not able to stretch my arms above my head, my back was crooked, my chest was tight and cramped. And yet I had always thought I was in pretty good shape for a guy of thirty.

I studied with Arthur Balaskas for about three years. We not only did yoga postures but also talked about the relationships of the joints, muscles and spine, which had the effect of allowing me to see the body as a whole system. We developed postures and exercises to 'loosen up' my body and I pursued them in a fairly disciplined fashion, exercising three to four hours per week. The result is that in some ways

I am looser than when I began. Whereas I could not touch my toes, I can now comfortably sit straight-legged on the floor with my chest flat on my legs. My progress has not been so remarkable in other postures. Nonetheless, my chest is no longer collapsed and I seem to stand straighter. But essentially, to me, this yoga 'feels right'. Sometimes I have to push myself to do an hour of exercises, but afterwards I am always glad that I did.

**David S. Goldblatt, psychotherapist**

One morning approximately three years ago, I awoke to discover I was beginning to live inside my father's body. There I was, twenty-five years old, eating pizza and ice cream all day, talking about my days as captain of the track team, as I drove my cumbersome mass the two blocks to the newspaper agent to pick up some cigarettes and candy. You might say vanity was my first step into yoga.

Even though I was vain in my attempt to regain youth lost, this did not mean I actually realized I had anything wrong with me. After all, I was training as a child psychotherapist (analytic) and my belief in mind over matter was at its peak; so, to change my shape, all I had to do was think about it. When there was pain, I ran to the specialist, acupuncturist, osteopath or homeopath, and it wasn't until I realized that most of this pain was tension, tension which I had locked inside myself, that I came to the conclusion that there wasn't going to be any potion to cure this illness. Through the process of my own analysis and practising certain movements, I began to separate what in fact was mental and what was physical.

I was overly strong, especially my neck and shoulders; somewhere in my mind I was still street-fighting. This was the hardest thing for me to break down. The idea that strength was health, that the stronger I was the healthier I was, had been embedded in my mind since a child. What I neglected to see was that force is a function of gravity; the more you struggle against it the more effort is required even to move. My problem was to strike a balance between relaxation and effort, forming a pose that used the natural forces which surrounded me at all times, and not to use myself in a way which was trying to overpower them. Eventually, by stretching and relaxing, I found I was beginning to discover my point of balance. As a result, my protruding eyes began to recede back into my head, headaches ceased, duck-footed feet began to point forward and in general I was becoming healthy, supple, and, in fact, to my surprise, stronger. By conserving energy, I seemed to have more strength without bulk.

**Robby Stein, child psychotherapist (clinical student)**

# 22 A look at yoga and meditation

## *Yoga*

The word 'yoga' literally means union or harmony. In its ultimate sense it means union with the unknown or absolute and any method of obtaining this. Each Eastern country has its version of yoga; for instance, there are Indian, Tibetan and Chinese yogas. Within each of these there are again many types aiming at the same goal but ·emphasizing different aspects. Indian or Hindu yoga alone encompasses Hatha Yoga (postures and rhythmic breath control), Mantra Yoga (repetition of sounds), Karma Yoga (work and action), Jnana Yoga (wisdom) and many more. Within each of these, too, because the methods have been passed down for centuries from teacher to pupil, there is again considerable variation. Each master or school has a particular version. But although the details vary the general structure is the same.

The great yoga classic of Sanskrit literature is the *Aphorisms* of Patanjali. He defines yoga as the stilling of the mind and lays down the method of attaining this in eight parts: (1) moral conduct, (2) self-purification, (3) posture, (4) rhythmic breath control, (5) withdrawal of the senses, (6) concentration, (7) meditation, and (8) super-consciousness. The theme of yoga by this method is control (male principle).

In the text 'posture' is defined as a firm and steady sitting position. Now this can be and has been interpreted in two different ways. On the one hand, it is taken merely to mean that one should find a comfortable position regardless of one's degree of flexibility, whether one is in good physical shape or not. On the other hand, it may mean that one should have a flexible body in very good physical condition in order to be able to sit firm and steady without disturbance or pain from one's body.

From the tradition of those who took the latter view have come the many yoga movements or postures. These movements used for the tempering of the body, plus the rhythmic breathing exercises and vegetarianism, have come to the West as popular yoga. Yoga proper requires a personal teacher or master and a specific way of life. It is a daily discipline demanding particular rules, behaviour and practices, including the non-use of meat, alcohol and tobacco. Yoga says 'If you do these things that Yogis have discovered you will eventually be free from suffering'.

I have always felt that it is presumptuous and impractical to lay down definite rules as to what we are to do. The theme of control and the way of life do not appeal to me, but the yoga movements do. I have adopted only those that accord with the common sense of modern anatomy. These I have studied and practised over the years, and through trial and error have reduced and modified them to the best advantage. From the rest of the system of yoga I have adopted very little.

Yoga, in its broadest sense, means 'skill in all activities', and any means of achieving this. Music, writing, art, dancing, and so on can all be seen as a yoga. In this sense, intelligent exercise that promotes flexibility, the ability to balance upside down and keen proprioception can also be called yoga.

The gymnastics of the early Greeks used similar positions and movements to those of yoga. Originally they were used for the development of the body and promotion of its efficiency, and therapeutically for many diseases and in the preparation of women for childbirth. However, gymnastics, which literally in the Greek means to train the body in the nude, has developed into a competitive sport and an artistic performance. In modern times movement and balance are cultivated mainly for this reason. The therapeutic aspect of gymnastics and its normal function of keeping the body in par condition have been forgotten or neglected.

Both yoga movements and gymnastics make use of extreme movements to temper the body. The point of yoga postures is to be able to sit still so that one becomes unconscious of the operations of the body, while gymnastics turns outwards into a display of the body's strength, flexibility, balance, speed, timing, control, and so on. In both disciplines the body is trained to fulfil its full potential for movement at every joint, and yet the aims of each could not, apparently, be more different.

But what about the simple purpose of developing an efficient, flexible, strong body, in order to promote full movement at the joints for its own sake? The purpose of the exercises in this book is just that, and the text preceding the exercises indicates both that it is possible and that the responsibility for achieving it is ours.

# Meditation

The 'awareness' (Satipatthāna) discourse of the Buddha is one of the earliest Pali texts, and considered by most Buddhists as the essence of their whole meditation practice. The ancient Greeks advised everyone 'to know themselves'. This text advises us to know ourselves *at every moment*. This is the crux of meditation.

According to the text, the only way to happiness and freedom from suffering is to apply awareness to four fundamentals: the body, sensations, emotions (feelings) and thinking (ideas). The key is the word 'awareness' and its meaning.

There is a basic difference between consciousness as a state of awareness and consciousness as a state of thinking. Thinking about something, a fact, for example, is a state of mind that goes round and round, a sort of internal dialogue. But awareness is a still point of consciousness, witnessing the evidence without any internal dialogue. It is a state of focused direction of the will between oneself as subject and one's chosen object, always in the here and now.

The text suggests that one apply this state of mind called awareness to everything that happens. Like all great techniques, it is simple, but like all great techniques it is masked by confused thinking. The implication here is that the ordinary everyday activities which one does repeatedly with awareness change one more effectively than anything else. Its essence is non-interference, merely witnessing whatever happens (feminine principle). No rules, commandments or specific way of life are required, no teacher or master. 'Be a lamp unto yourself' is the theme. It is a matter of applying awareness at all times, of meditation in action, a training of the mind. Meditation as a particular exercise done in a formal way, is simply the ritual enjoyment of this basic awareness of what is happening from moment to moment. The good of awareness is awareness, not some result it may bring.

The text suggests a treatment of the four fundamentals; the body, sensations, emotions and thinking. The only reference to actually sitting down is in the very first instruction on awareness of breathing. It says: 'Having gone to the forest, to the foot of a tree or to an empty place, one sits down cross-legged, keeps one's body erect and one's awareness alert. Just with awareness one breathes in and breathes out.'

We don't know what physical shape the people Buddha addressed were in, but for most of us sitting down for any length of time with legs crossed and body erect is a tall order. Again, as in the definition of posture by Patanjali, merely sitting in any comfortable position may be all that is meant; but I take it as implying that one's body must be so flexible and in such shape that one can sit cross-legged with body erect.

Awareness of the duration of one's breathing is an exercise in awareness and not a breathing exercise like the breath control (pranayama) of Hindu yoga. There is no control or retention of breath or any interference with it. There is just a quiet *attention* to its natural flow. The length or shortness of breathing is noticed, but not deliberately regulated. Regular practice, however, will result quite naturally in a calming and deepening of the breath.

In the section on the body, after breathing as an object of awareness, come the positions of the body. One should be fully aware when going, standing, sitting or lying down or in any position of the body. One should be 'clearly conscious in going and coming, in looking forward and backward, in bending and stretching, in eating, drinking, speaking, keeping silent', and so on. At this point, the text suggests that one reflect on (1) the contents of the body, that one is made of blood, flesh, bones, mucus, and so on, (2) the material elements of the body, the earth, water, fire and air elements, and (3) that the body cannot escape death, and that this is part of its nature. I have found that by cultivating movement and keener proprioception one automatically and effortlessly improves one's awareness of any position of one's body and that the best time to reflect on the nature of one's body, as suggested by the text, is while practising self-massage.

Intelligent exercise that promotes flexibility, the ability to balance upside down and proprioceptive sensation and aliveness is to me not merely a frill but a basic human need. For thousands of years, many religions and disciplines have deemed the tempering of the body the first step towards freeing the mind and spirit. Modern teachers, too, stress the essentiality of this. Krishnamurti says:

'We are concerned not only with the cultivation of the mind and the awakening of emotional sensitivity, but also a well-rounded development of the physique, and so to this we must give considerable thought. For if the body is not healthy, vital, it will inevitably distort thought and make for insensitivity. This is so obvious that we need not go into it in detail. It is necessary that the body be in excellent health, that it be given the right kind of food and have sufficient sleep. If the senses are not alert, the body will impede the whole development of the human being. To have grace of movement and well-balanced control of the muscles, there must be various forms of exercise, dancing and games. A body that is not kept clean, that is sloppy and does not hold itself in good posture, is not conducive to sensitivity of mind and emotions. The body is not the instrument of the mind, but body [movement and sensation] emotions and mind make up the total human being, and unless they live together harmoniously, conflict is inevitable.'

And as Lao-Tzu put it two thousand years ago:

> 'Man at his birth is supple and tender
> But in death he is rigid and hard
> Now plants when young are sinuous and moist
> But when old are brittle and dry.
> Thus suppleness and tenderness are signs of life,
> While rigidity and hardness are signs of death.'

# Index

Abdominal exercises, 114–15
Achilles tendon, exercise, 124
Ankle joints, 40
    order for exercising, 141
    relaxing, 57
Arches, falling, 43
Arms, balancing on elbows,
    136–7
    description, 33
    exercises with, 64, 65–6, 181
    joints, 38–9
    movements, 38–9
    relaxing, 55
    stretching sideways, 65–6
Arthritis, 41

Back, see Backbone
Backache, exercises for, 166–76
Backbone, description, 31–2
    in pregnancy, 160, 164
    limitations of, 36–7
    order for exercising, 142–3
    relaxing, 55
Backward bending, 36–7
    exercises, 110–13
Balance and relaxing, 58
    building up, 46
    seat of, 13
Blood system, 47–9
Boat position, 114, 153
Body, awareness, see Exercises,
    muscle; Proprioception
    building up, 46
    knowing your own, 11–16,
        20–9
        description, 11–16
        facial parts, 22–3
        hands, using, 20–1
        head massage, 23–9
        massage, 21–2
        temperature, 49
Bones, 30–3
Breathing, 48, 50–2, 61

Camel position, 112, 151
Cartilages, 34
Chest and breathing, 50–2
    description, 32, 37
    joints in, 39
Children, exercises for and with,
    150–8:
    boat position, 153
    butterfly position, 153
    camel position, 151
    cobra position, 152
    crab position, 155
    dog position, 152
    elbow stand, 155
    fish position, 152
    frog position, 151
    handstand, 154
    headstand, 158
    jack-knife position, 153
    lion position, 157
    lotus position, 156
    plough position, 152
    rabbit position, 157
    seal position, 152
    sitting easy, 150
    sloth position, 152
    splits, 155
    tailor position, 156
    tortoise position, 151
    tree position, 153
Chin, massaging, 21
Circulation of blood, 47
Cobra position, 113, 152
Collarbones, 32, 37
    see also Shoulders
Crab position, 112, 155

Diaphragm, 51–2
Discs, slipped, 34
Disjointedness, 41
Dog position, 90, 113, 152

Ears, massaging, 28
Elbows, balancing on, 136–7, 155

Equipment needed, 59–60
Exercises:
    children's, see Children
    for backache, 166–76
    for balance, 125–38:
        elbow, 136–7
        hands, 138
        head, 131–6
        neck, 126–31
        shoulder, 126–31
    in the office, 178–83
    muscle:
        (for) abdominal, 114–15
        achilles tendon, 124
        arms, 64–6, 116–19
        backward bending, 110–13
        back bending, 110–13
        boat position, 114
        camel position, 112
        cobra position, 113
        crab position, 112
        dog position, 90, 113
        feet, 120–1
        hamstrings, 76, 102
        hands, 67
        head, 62–3
        legs extended, feet together,
            94–5
            feet apart, 96–9
        lotus position, 105–6
        martial stance, 81–8
        neck, 62–3
        on back, feet apart, knees
            together, 106
        on one leg, 79
        pelvis, 68–70, 73, 74
        sitting between feet, 100–2
        splits, 99–104
        squatting, 87–9
        standing, 68–70
        tailor position, 92–3
        ten most important, list of,
            107
        toes, 122–4
        trunk, extending, 110–13
            rotating, 80
            sideways, 77–8
            twisting, 108–9
        wrist, 119
        see also under Children
    rules for, 59–61
    with others, 144–9
Eyes and eyebrows, massaging, 24

Face, massaging, 22–9
Fatigue, overcoming, 53
Feet, exercises for, 101–2, 120–1
    joints in, 40
    order of exercising, 143
    relaxing, 57
    when pregnant, 159
Flat-footedness, 43
Flexibility, 62–7
Footwear, suitable, 121–2
Forehead, massaging, 23
Friction and massage, 21

Gravity and:
    balance, 125–38
    heart action, 47–8
    muscle power, 45

Hamstrings, 56
    exercises, 76, 102, 179–80
Hands:
    balancing on, 138
    exercises using, 67, 138
    magic touch of, 20
    movements, 39
    order for exercising, 143
    -stand (children), 154
Head:
    balance exercises for, 131–6
    joints in, 35
    office exercises for, 182
    relaxing, 54–5
    -stand (children), 158
Heart action, 47–9
Heels, sitting on, when pregnant,
    161–3

Hips:
    and backache, 173–6
    bones in, 33
    load on, 39–40
    order for exercising, 141
    relaxing, 56
    see also Pelvis

Jack-knife position, 153
Joints of the body, 34–41:
    backbone limitations, 36–7
    disjointedness, 41
    hips, load on, 39–40
    in the arm, 38–9
    in the chest, 39
    in the leg, 40
    neck, 36
    shoulders, 37
    universal, 35
    using the right ones, 34–5

Kneading, 20–1
Knees:
    joints of, 40
    order for exercising, 141

Legs:
    exercises for, 79, 94–9
    joints in, 40
    relaxing, 55, 57
    shape of, 15
    skeleton of, 33
Ligaments, 43
Limbs, see Arms, Legs
Lotus position, 105–6, 156
Lungs:
    and breathing, 50–2
    oxygen needs for, 44
Lymph, 49

Marrow, bone, 33
Martial stance, 81–6
Massage:
    and pregnancy, 159
    in general, 20–2
    of face and head, 23–9
    types of, 21
Medical examinations, 42
Meditation and yoga, 188–91
Menstruation and exercises, 59
Movements:
    and muscles, 42–3
    and pain, 60–1
    of joints, 34–5
    order for exercise, 140–3
    rules for, 59–61
    three categories of, 12–13
    time to be spent on, 60
    when pregnant, 160–5:
        for pelvis, 165
        lying down, 165
        on back, 164
        on heels, 161–3
        squatting, 160
        tailor position, 161
Muscles:
    and breathing, 51
    and will-power, 14–15
    fibres, 43
    four classes of, 44–5
    intercostal, 51
    matters in general, 42–6:
        body building through, 46
        gravity and, 45
        involuntary, 42–3
        ligaments, 43
        mechanics of, 44
        power of, 42
        tendons, 43
        voluntary, 42–3
        what they do, 44–5
    of the skin, 43
    relaxing, 53–8
    see also Relaxing

Neck:
    and backache, 169–72
    and flexibility, 62–3, 182
    balance exercises for, 126–31
    joints in, 36

office exercises for, 182
    order for exercising, 140
    relaxing, 54–5
Nose and massage, 24–5

Office, exercising in the, 178–83:
    arm rotation, 181
    hamstrings, 179–80
    head, 182–3
    neck, 182
    sitting positions, 183
    squatting, 179
Oxygen needs, 44

Pain:
    exercises and, 60–1
    friends with, 17–19:
        overcoming suffering, 17–18
        seats of, 12
        what is beneficial and what
            harmful, 18–19
Pelvis:
    and breathing, 52
    description, 33
    exercises for, 68–70,73,74, 167–8
        when pregnant, 165
    relaxing, 56
    see also Hips
Plough position, 145, 152
Pregnant condition, 159–65
Proprioception, 13–16, 42, 59

Relaxing, 53–8:
    ankles and legs, 57
    backbone, 55
    hips, 56
    neck and head, 54–5
    shoulders, 55
Resting exercises, 139
Ribs, 32
Rules for movement, 59–61

Safety limits, 59
Scalp, massaging, 29
Seal position, 152
Self-confidence, gaining, 15–16
Shoes, suitable, 121–2
Shoulders:
    and backache, 169–72
    balance exercises for, 126–31
    description, 32, 37
    joints in, 37
    order for exercising, 140
    relaxing, 55
Sitting position (in offices), 183
Skeleton, 30–3
Skin, appearance of, 20
Skull, description, 31
Sleeping, positions for, 177
Spine, see Backbone
Splits, 99, 104, 155
Squatting exercise, 87–9, 145, 160, 179
Standing exercises, 68–70
Stroking in massage, 21
Synovial fluid and joints, 34–5

Tailor position, 92–3, 156, 161
Temperature, maintaining body, 49
Tendons, 43
Tenseness, see Relaxing
Testimonials, 184–7
Thighs, see Hips; Pelvis
Throat massage, 28
Toe exercises, 122–4
Tree position, 153
Trunk exercises, 68–70, 77–8, 80, 108–9, 110–13

Vertebrae, five groups of, 31

Warmth, maintaining body, 49
Weight:
    and the skeleton, 30–1
    shifting the centre of, by body
        movements, 41
Will-power, 14–15
Wrists:
    exercises for, 119
    order for exercising, 143

Yoga and meditation, 188–91